Frank Riley with Words from Danny Riley

Sit and Listen: Reflections of a Father and Son

Danny Riley Music
www.dannyriley.com

"A Blessing" by John O'Donohue, from **Eternal Echoes: Celtic Reflections On Our Yearning to Belong,** and excerpt from **Anam Cara: A Book of Celtic Wisdom** reproduced with kind permission from John's family and Perennial, An Imprint of Harper Collins Publishers.

"The Strength of Others," by Fr. William Atkinson, OSA, www.fatherbillatkinson.org, reproduced with kind permission of the Atkinson family. Excerpt from "**Till Death Do Us Part,"** reproduced with permission of author Phil Coulter.

Excerpts from **OUR APPOINTMENT with LIFE: Discourse on Living Happily in the Present Moment,** by Thich Nhat Hanh, Parallax Press, Berkeley, California, www.parallax.org and **The Reasons of Love** by Harry G. Frankfurt, University of Pittsburg Press, reproduced with permission of publishers.

Danny Riley's words and poems were on his laptop or in his journal, as he wrote them, unedited.

Covers designed by Francisco Franco.
Back cover photo taken by Alicia Riley.

In Loving Memory of Daniel Joseph Riley and those in his circle of love who have passed away:

Betty Baker, Danny's grandmother who died with Danny at her side two months before his brain tumor was discovered.

Joe Osborn, aka Papa Joe, Danny's uncle, surrogate paternal grandfather, who passed away a few months before Danny's diagnosis.

Edward Riley, Danny's uncle, who was by his side for his first surgery and a trip home from Santa Barbara, full of Ed's real life stories.

Kathleen Connell, Danny's, full of antics but loving, aunt.

Fr. Bill Atkinson, O.S.A., family friend and an inspiration to Danny.

Barbara Arvin, Danny's uncle Darryl's sister, who always made him laugh.

Jeff Johnson, Jack's dad, who shared Danny's love of the ocean.

Mickey Nickens, Danny's cousin Karen's husband, who like Danny was a big sports fan.

Beau Lamar, Danny's cousin Kate's husband, who shared Danny's passion for music.

Gordon Baker, Danny's grandfather who died at age 95, but at 91 said goodbye to his youngest grandchild.

Rosemarie Osborn, aka Nana Rose, Danny's aunt who was like his grandmother lived clos to Riley family until Danny's diagnosis in 2004.Manny pictures on Nana Rose in the book.

Tom Riley, Danny's uncle, whose home in Philadelphia Danny visited many times and enjoyed Uncle Tom's stories and humor.

Don Baker, Danny's great uncle, whose San Francisco Home and knowledge of the city Danny enjoyed.

Sheila Brucelas, Danny's "sister" trough the bonds of family forged by her mother Toni starting when she lived as a teenager with the Baker family Danny and Sheila was as close as blood relatives. Like Danny, Sheila had a smile and warmth that could light-up a room and died too young.

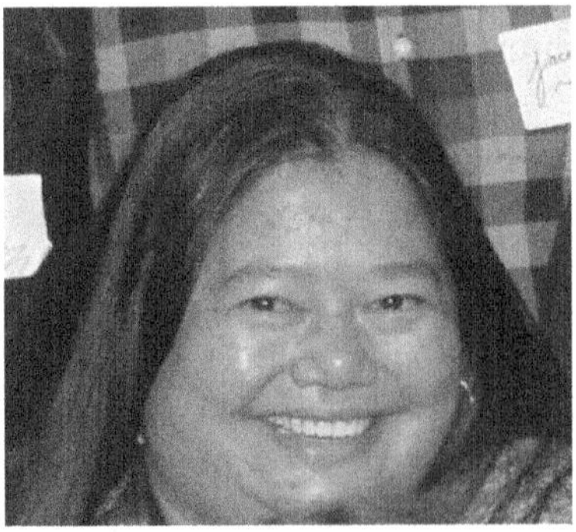

A Blessing

May you know that absence is full of tender presence and that nothing is ever lost or forgotten.

May the absences in your life be full of eternal echo.

May you sense around you the secret Elsewhere which holds the presences that have left your life.

May you be generous in your embrace of loss.

May the sore well of grief turn into a well of seamless presence.

May your compassion reach out to the ones we never hear from and may you have the courage to speak out for the excluded ones.

May you become the gracious and passionate subject of your own life.

May you not disrespect your mystery through brittle words or false belonging.

May you be embraced by God in whom dawn and twilight are one, and may your belonging inhabit its deepest dreams within the shelter of the Great Belonging.

-John O'Donohue

Contents

Build-Up

The following pages tell pieces of a story. Many of the words are those of my late son Danny, others are my own reflections about his life, and some are the connections needed to weave a good story. I come from a large family of Irish descent, so story-telling is part of our heritage. My dad loved a good story and told many of his own. When one of us shared something bad that happened to us, his reply would usually be: "Well, at least, you got a story out of it!"

This story is sparked by the life of my son Danny that ended on October 31, 2007, as a result of brain cancer. When he died he was almost twenty. If you are like my dad, who did not like to hear sad news and would switch to the topic: "How are the Phillies (baseball team) doing?" you may not want to go further, thinking it will be too sad. If you do, you will miss out on a good story. Certainly sadness runs through it, but I hope that in reading Danny's words you will see that his own life, even to the last breaths, was not filled with sadness. He let others and his inner life fill it with love and hope. He left many words on his laptop, beacons that shine light on the journey.

One note stands out and is the backdrop of this tale:

> **when im dead**
> **and they write about me in retrospect**
> **i dont want the writing to be about**
> **my acomplishments**
> **but rather**
> **my loves.**
> **all those that i have loved**
> **and all those that have loved me.**

This story will be true to this wish because Danny's accompishments were his loves: all those he loved and who loved him. He sang about them, smiled, shared his pain and joy with them, and died surrounded by those he loved and who loved him. While I am the narrrator, I am not alone in the telling of it. Danny's mother and my wife, Maggi and his sister Alicia, who make up ***Team Danny***, helped me along with others in this "labor of love." This is about people, pain, and the power of loving relationships: family, friends, caregivers, all who were campanions on Danny's journey. You are asked to join by reading and seeing pictures about our travels with him and each other. Hopefully, this will be a "good story," inspiring you to appreciate and share the stories life's joys and sorrows inspire.

Frank Riley
Chula Vista, California
October, 2011, Revised September, 2019

1
The Beginning

Amid the rush of our lives, it is easy to miss the meaning, the gifts of life's fleeting moments. Such a statement is certainly not new. It is a theme that is woven throughout history. While Danny's story touches on this, it does not ask anything of you but to stop and listen to his reflections. His struggle sparked my own writing about the gifts of his life and death. You are asked to take a journey that may be sad at times but may also be uplifting and inspiring.

"Sit and Listen" is the title of one of Danny's songs. He wrote and recorded this song on his laptop sometime between December 2004, when he was diagnosed with brain cancer, and October 31, 2007, the day he died at age 19. The lyrics tell of his inward journey:

> I sit and I listen
> to all that you enter
> while praying in silence
> …Memory fills me
> therefore I see blindly.
> The task is uncertain
> and so is its meaning....
> But what we don't notice
> is that it's really inside.
> As I sing this, it pauses
> to breathe in the spirit

the treasures around us:
the world and its people.
So if there is goodness
please pay us a visit.
The path is uncertain.
Please help us to find it…

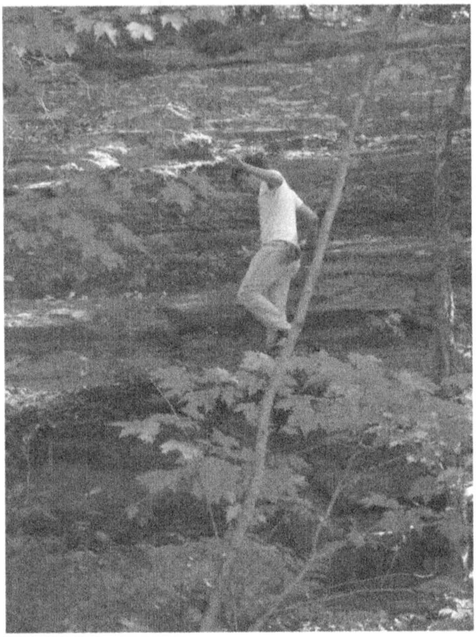

Danny's uncertain path was full of people who helped him find his way, but his real guide came from within, as we will see as we travel with him. Danny's was born on December 12, 1987, but our story begins on December 8, 2004. Here's how Danny described that day:

It cannot be expressed in words, but I will do my best to share a part of myself with you. This is the story of the greatest experience of my life.

I have always been a thoughtful individual, with many desires and passions. Education has always been a way for me to better myself as a person and enrich my life through engaging my mind. Over a year ago, as I entered my junior year in high school, I was just starting to get a better sense of myself as an adolescent. Then it happened: the headaches.

I would describe the utterly blinding and crippling pain for you in full detail, although, I have blocked out most of my memories of the experience. They started on Saturday night, waking me up from a peaceful and much needed sleep. My mother consoled and tended me as best she could, but the agony persisted through the night and into the next morning. I'd never had serious headaches before, so we all just assumed it was a temporary migraine, probably brought on by over exertion at school and soccer (my mom always warned me about doing headers.). I took some Tylenol, but the pain pressed on through the day. By Sunday night it seemed much worse. I felt nauseated and vomited up what little food was in my stomach. At the same time I noticed some of my fingers were going numb with a strange tingling sensation. As has always been my best defense, I tried to laugh it all off, and soothe my pain away with deep breathing. My mom, dad, and I had all decided that I should stay home from school the next day. Monday came around and my dad stayed home from work to be with me. I was feeling much better during the day, and my dad and I had some fun being lazy hanging around the house. The day was bright and warm, and I began to forget that I had ever felt bad at all. That night I made up some of my uncompleted homework and slept beautifully.

School the next day was a bit of a blur. Mildly concerned friends wondering where I had been the previous day were matched by a nice amount of work I had missed out on. I played left defense in the varsity soccer game late that afternoon, drove home and crashed out on the couch for an immediate nap. I woke up for some dinner and homework, and then went to bed.

That night at 4 o'clock it hit. The headache came back with relentless waves of terrible pain. By this time we needed to figure out a way to make the pain stop so I could get on with school and such. Wednesday morning, my mom and dad took me to the doctor to get some medication to keep the pain down.

At first I was met by a student doctor who diligently examined every bit of me that could possibly be involved with my mysterious headaches. Then a very wise and regal looking doctor with a snowy white beard entered the room and effortlessly examined me while his student gave his report. I explained what had happened to him slowly and carefully. He seemed about ready to prescribe some routine painkillers, when my mother remembered to mention how my fingers had gone numb during the headaches. I showed him which ones and he reassuringly suggested that I have a CAT-SCAN just to make sure it's nothing serious. He had such a warm and benign aura that we were all certain that nothing was at all the matter with me, but it's just good to get proof.

My mom left for work and my dad hung around with me to get the CAT-SCAN over with. I was excited about it. It was absolutely intriguing for me to find out what this scan was like. They laid me down on the table, strapped my head in place, and slide me back. It wasn't the scary, dark hole that I had envisioned but more like a loud, techno donut. The only bad part was when they injected some contrast into my arm (I hated needles.). It lasted for a good 30 minutes and after, we slouched down in the waiting room. That's when it hit: the heartache.

“Mr. Riley... We are going to send you up to admittance. A doctor will meet you there.” I vaguely knew what that meant, but nothing in me said it was going to be a bad thing. Dad knew it could only mean bad news. As we walked up to the admittance building, my father held me tight against him. I tried to console him. We walked with arms over each other’s shoulders. The clerk told us to take a seat. As we did, a familiar face walked towards us. It was my pediatrician, Dr. McQuaide. He greeted us with a deep affectionate smile. ”Let’s go have some privacy.” He led us to a small consult room. We sat down and everyone took a deep quivering breath of air. He wasted no time with pleasantries and got straight to the point.

“The CAT-SCAN showed a tumor in the right frontal lobe of Danny’s brain.”
The news came as a terrible shock to my father, but I listened intently with my eyes fixed on Dr. McQuaide, briskly nodding my head up and down as if I knew what he was talking about. Dr. McQuaide proceeded to explain that I was to be held overnight in the hospital so they could take some more scans and tests. He took us out of the room and

> explained to the nurse at the counter that I was to be admitted. "What is he to be admitted for?" the nurse asked politely. I watched as Dr. McQuaide tried to say 'brain tumor' but couldn't quite muster the heart to do it. Instead, he dropped his eyes, scribbled something down on a piece of paper, and slid it towards the nurse. The nurse asked us to have a seat until we were called. Dr. McQuaide said he would come visit me later that day.
>
> Once again we sat in the waiting room. Dad leaned over towards me. With glossy eyes and a voice full of trembling pride he said, "You'll be our Lance Armstrong. You'll beat it." "I know," I thought to myself.

While most stories don't begin with the outcome, you already know Danny's. He did not "beat it," but he certainly tried: living fully and courageously, singing and smiling, gathering others to share his inspiring journey to live a normal life with brain cancer. This excerpt from an essay he wrote in the fall of 2005 for his application to various campuses of the University of California shows this spirit:

> ...A year ago, I had a craniotomy to remove a four-and-a-half by five-centimeter malignant tumor from my brain. The surgery went well, but that's not really the hard part in my opinion; all I had to do was fall asleep. Because of the high grade of my

cancer, I have doubled up with both radiation and chemotherapy to best counteract any tumor recurrence. The semester after my surgery, I had to take Incompletes in Physics and AP Calculus, which I later made up, and drop two of my classes to make time for radiation therapy. What might seem like an ominous, daily trek downtown to a facility full of the walking dead soon became a lovely ritual. I felt a great deal of pride and humor in being the youngest person at the radiation center, by about forty to fifty years. I also took it as my obligation to bring some youthful spirit into a place so drenched in mourning, with maybe just a simple smile or a pleasant comment. It comforted me as much as it comforted all the other patients, sitting alone in that waiting room filled with nervous glances and outdated magazines.

Because of my treatment I do miss out on school when I'm feeling sick or have appointments. Also, the effects of the treatment make it difficult to play sports as I once did. But I have learned to overcome these barriers, as they cannot stop me from living a normal life. Living a normal life: that is one of my proudest achievements. Despite everything that has happened to me, I know that I am still able to do anything I set my mind to. Whether it be working diligently in school and ASB, enjoying music, or being there for my friends and family, I can still live life to the fullest.

Having brain cancer is the greatest thing that has happened to me. It has given me a new life as opposed to taking one away. This concept may be hard to grasp, but I have begun to appreciate everything with fresh insight now that I have seen how life can be cut short, both in years and quality. With this comes a stronger appreciation of the friends and family that have helped me throughout.

I don't remember myself before cancer, and I don't think it's because they accidentally took that part of my brain out with the tumor. Instead, it is because I am happy as who I am today. I don't miss being cancer-free and I wouldn't trade the world to have my life be any other way than it is right now, brain cancer and all. I'm a better person than I was before. I can adapt, I can appreciate, and I can love on a whole different level than before. What I may lack in energy at times, I make up for with an enhancement of my connection with life and the present moment. And whatever time I may lose out on in the future, I am sure to make up for by living now.

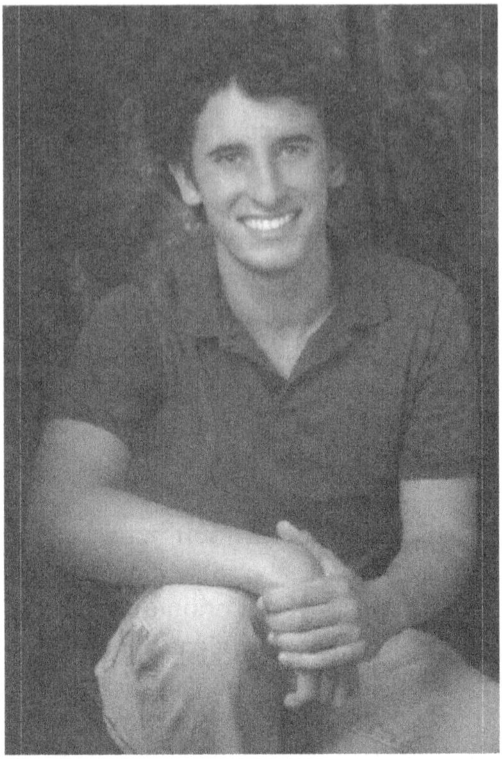

Danny's senior picture, fall, 2005

Danny was accepted at all the universities he applied to, and chose to go to the University of California at Santa Barbara. During his junior and most of his senior year of high school, Danny was treated with an oral chemo agent called Temodar. He took it for one week a month, which almost brought him to his knees by Thursday, but he was strong again by the weekend. He went through six weeks of radiation, as described above, and had MRIs every two months. These were intense times for all of us as we waited for the results. "The tumor is stable" were welcome words. However, the January 2006 MRI did not bring those words. There was growth and a new lesion on the right side of his brain. We had the new tumor treated with stereotactic radiation surgery. This was performed at Kaiser in Los Angeles and required that Danny's head have a brace attached that would fit into the equipment. The picture below shows him trying to smile through it:

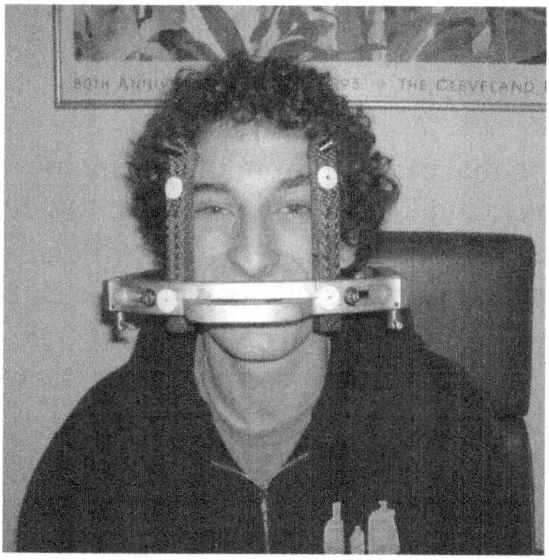

Danny had a good voice, learned to play the guitar and was writing songs; so, before we had the treatment, Danny's godfather Joe Dibos arranged for a two-day recording session on the weekend. Two days later we were off to Los Angeles and Danny was a great sport about it.

Danny subsequently entered a clinical trial conducted by the UCSF Medical Center in May of 2006. At first it showed promise, but by August the lesion on the side was growing again. Before he went to college, Danny had a portal cathedra put in his chest so he could get the new chemo agents without all the hand and arm pokes. To protect the placement of the port, doctors told him he should not play basketball, but, as I can attest, he continued to play. I will never forget the words of one of Danny's nurses at the time. He said that he hoped this would not happen, but the port was very helpful in administering pain medication for some of his young patients at the end of their lives. Again, as I can attest, this proved to be true for Danny.

A question that came up from the beginning was how Danny could be so positive in the face of such challenges? While the answer may be illusive, it is not unique to Danny, as others who have cared for or treated children or young adults with serious illnesses know. What may be unique to Danny is that he left his words and songs as a living testament to his quest to live fully, despite his struggle with brain cancer.

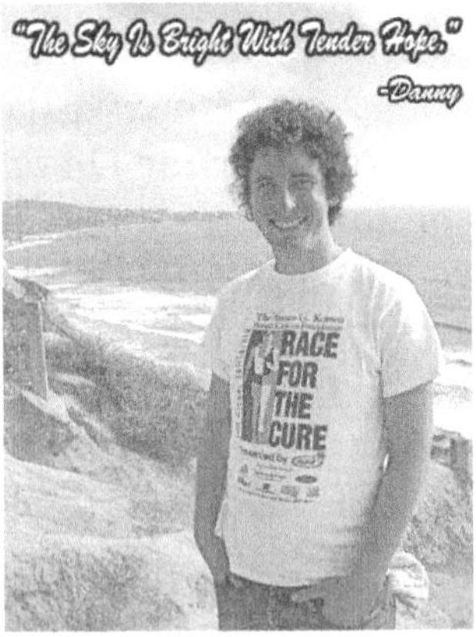

2
That's My Boy!

After he died, we found many poems, notes, songs on his laptop and in his journal. A couple of entries in his journal capture my Danny Boy in a powerful way. One poem "To Be Tender" expresses Danny's spirit and, at the same time, presents a challenge to us as we face our own difficulties.

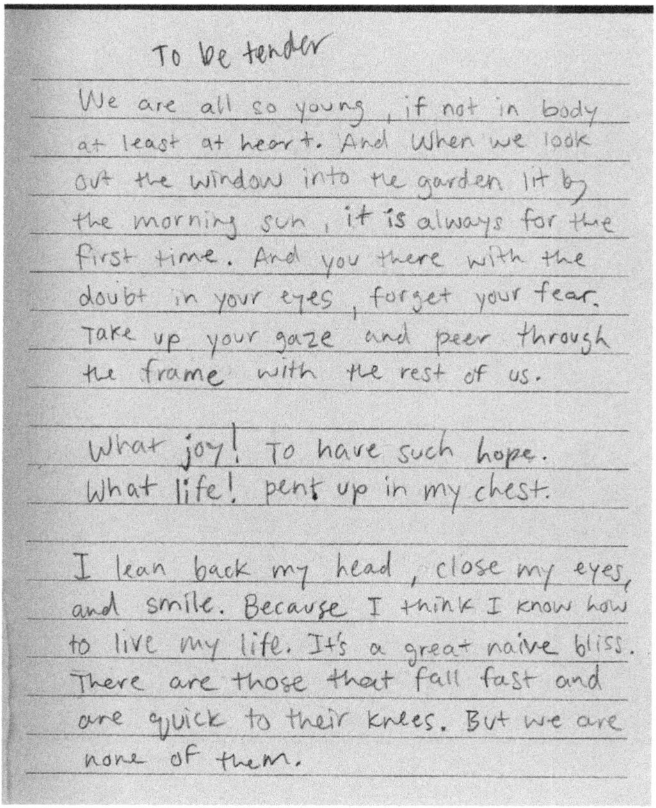

To be tender

We are all so young, if not in body at least at heart. And when we look out the window into the garden lit by the morning sun, it is always for the first time. And you there with the doubt in your eyes, forget your fear. Take up your gaze and peer through the frame with the rest of us.

What joy! To have such hope.
What life! pent up in my chest.

I lean back my head, close my eyes, and smile. Because I think I know how to live my life. It's a great naive bliss. There are those that fall fast and are quick to their knees. But we are none of them.

Artistic rendering by his life-long friend Sam Julian

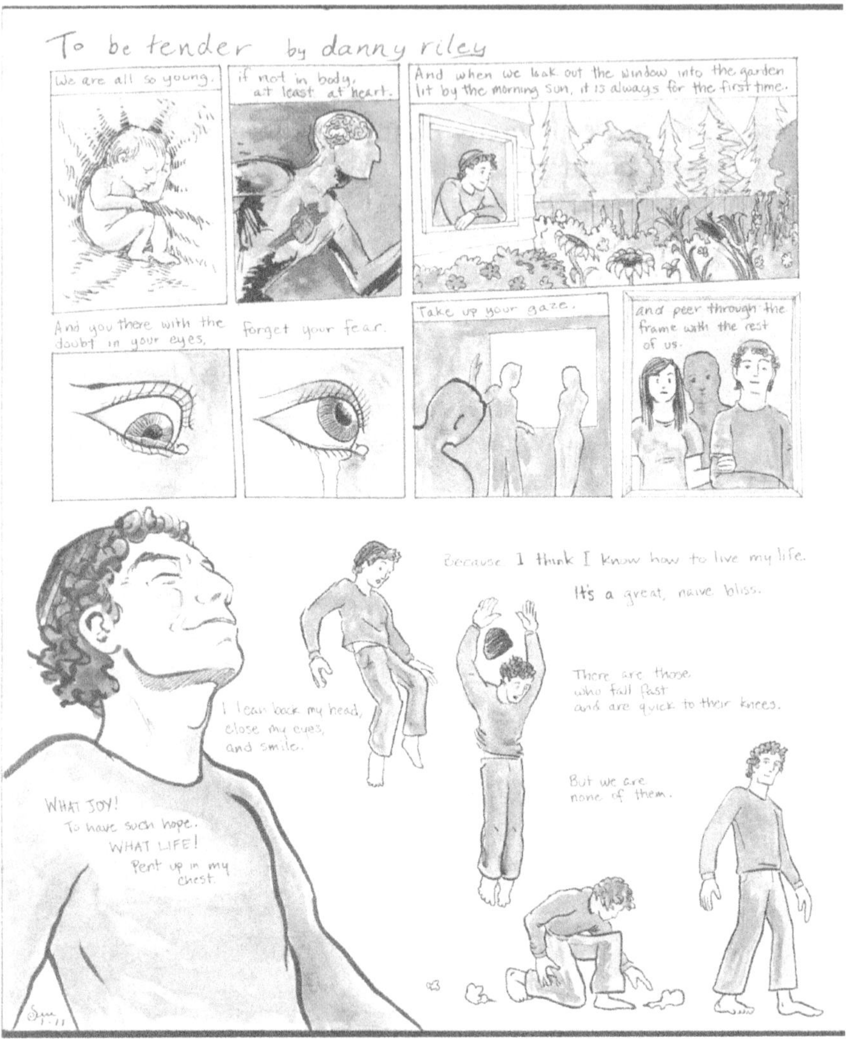

Another journal entry shows Danny's view of life:

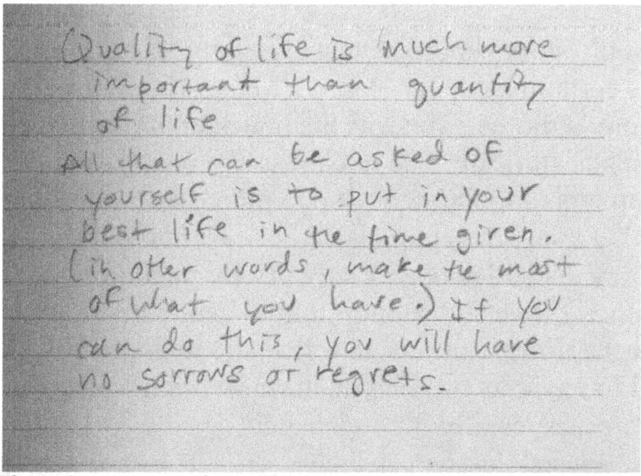
Quality of life is much more
important than quantity
of life
All that can be asked of
yourself is to put in your
best life in the time given.
(in other words, make the most
of what you have.) If you
can do this, you will have
no sorrows or regrets.

There's a part of me that wants to stop the story here with a big "That's my boy!" But the words and lyrics of Danny's journal entries and songs go on to elaborate how he overcame his fear and helped others to do the same. Once he asked me: "Poppy, how are you doing?" I replied that I was okay but worried about him. Danny quickly replied: "Do you see me worrying?" "No," I said. With reassurance in his voice, he quipped: "Follow my lead." We will see how he led as the story continues.

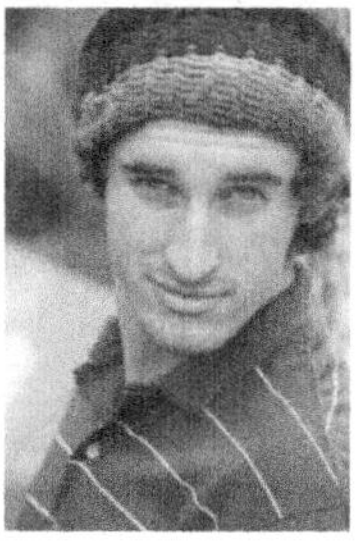 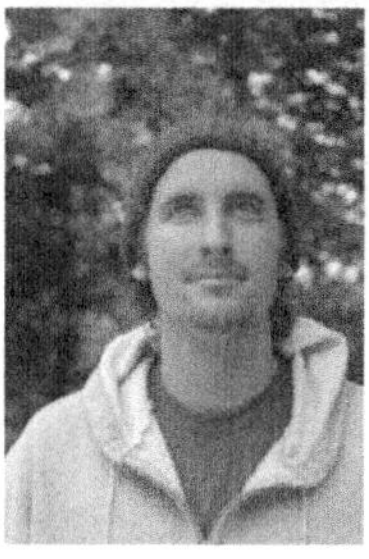

3
Mother and Health Care Manager

A son's story should have a caring mother and this was certainly true for Danny. Maggi is not only Danny's mother; she was the manager and overseer of his health care. She tracked every medication, treatment, appointment, and explored every option for her son, who appreciated her care and concern. Danny depended on her not only for unconditional motherly love and support, but to deal with the side effects of medications, to follow-up with doctors, and to navigate through the turmoil brain cancer creates, especially for a teenager.

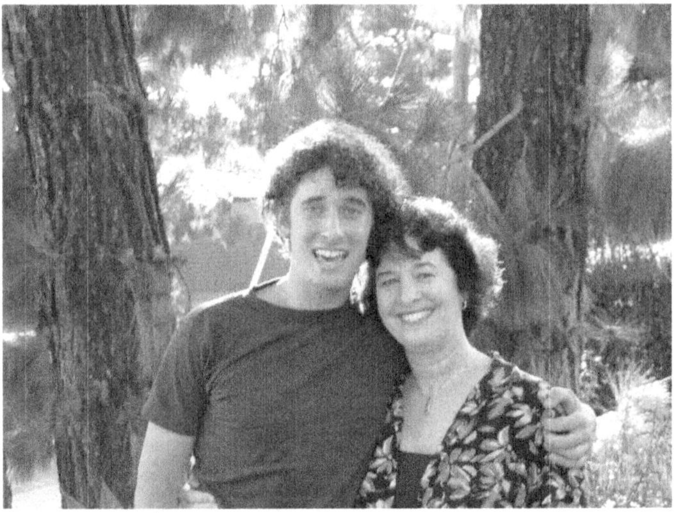

Danny's 2006 Mother's Day message is a beautiful tribute of his love for his mother:

Mom,

This is an attempt at just a few words,
Which might cause a smile or a warmth unheard
To convey pure love is my goal
To convey the spot which inside my soul
I cherish everything that you give to me,
In kindness, in sickness, and in tragedy.

I wish that you know, that within my heart,
Lies a bond of spirit, which you are a part.
To give your reflection, I truly must say
That God must have made you in a precious way.
For you are the one who can quell my fears,
And remain by my side through the darkest of years.

Your reflection is soft, and sweet as warm dew,
Your knowledge is deep, with wisdom and truth,
Your vision is clear, robust, and intact,
Your intentions are strong, hard-willed, and in contrast
With everything in this world of ours,
Which dampens the spirit and darkens the flowers.
I need you to know that I've already been blessed,

By having the greatest mother, surpassing all the rest.
For I don't believe that they could garnish the same love,
Or the resonating warmth of peace, which fills my heart and soul,
That you give to me.

And for that, I am forever your son,
With love and kindness,
I am always your one.

Love,
Danny

While Maggi assumed the role of the Health Care Manager for Danny's treatments, and is a professional in health promotion with a Doctorate in Public Health, she is and will always be first and foremost his mother. The intersection of the love of a mother and anguish at her son having brain cancer set her in motion to get him the best possible care. From the day of his diagnosis, she began researching treatment options, calling doctors at Duke, San Francisco, and other centers, known for treating brain tumors. She obtained approval from Kaiser Permanente, our family's health care provider, to have consultations with the UCSF Brain Tumor Center, paid for by Kaiser. However, her initial request for ongoing consultations from UCSF Brain Tumor Center was denied because they had too many patients. Undaunted, Maggi wrote an impassioned letter to them pleading that they take on Danny's case. Dr. Anu Banerjee, a pediatric neuro-oncologist, and a mother herself, accepted Danny's case and in so doing became a beacon of hope for him and our family. In the fall of 2005, Maggi was able to enroll in Blue Cross through her work, so we had dual coverage and were able to have actual treatments, including two surgeries, at UCSF Medical Center.

Danny used to say that when he was with Dr. Banerjee, he felt she was trying everything to have him survive and thrive, to live his dream of leading a normal life with brain cancer. She was always exploring clinical trials and in the late spring of 2006 during his senior year of high school he was accepted into a trial that she led. This required him to fly to San Francisco once a week for the first month of the trial, then once a month for the following three months that the experimental drug, Lapatinib, appeared to be working. Unfortunately, in August it stopped being effective. Dr. Banerjee used to say that clinical trials were like going for the home run. Well, we never got one over the fence, but we kept swinging for one.

While all doctors have to be somewhat detached from their patients, especially those treating younger ones with cancer, Danny's personality and wit made that difficult. He just connected with those caring for him, especially Dr. Banerjee. In between visits, we would have phone consultations, sort-of strategy sessions. Danny would always end on a positive note of appreciation.

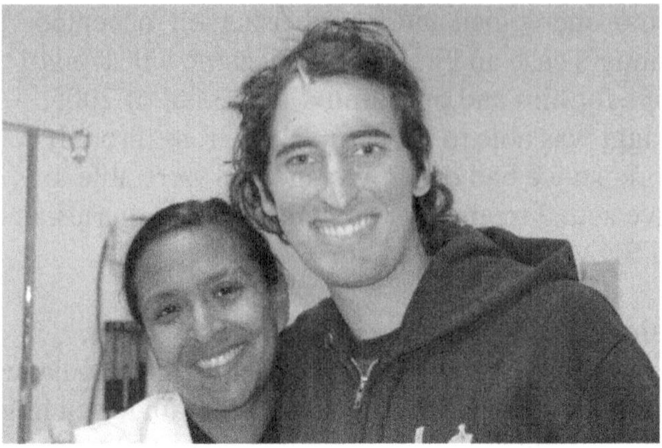

While Danny always found hope in his visits with Dr. Banerjee, our last consultation in late August 2007 was rough. The one word I remember she used to describe the situation was “dire.” Danny listened, asked questions, and voiced his usual appreciation, but it was a somber session. After it was over, Danny’s sister Alicia rose to the occasion with her own encouragement and support for Danny, telling him there is always hope.

4
Big Sister

Danny's story has a loving sister Alicia, who is two years older. She was his unspoken strength and confidant throughout his struggle with cancer. She helped him live his dream of a normal life. Danny was able to live, even smile, through his struggles because Alicia was with him, either by his side or calling him with her encouragement and lovingly support.

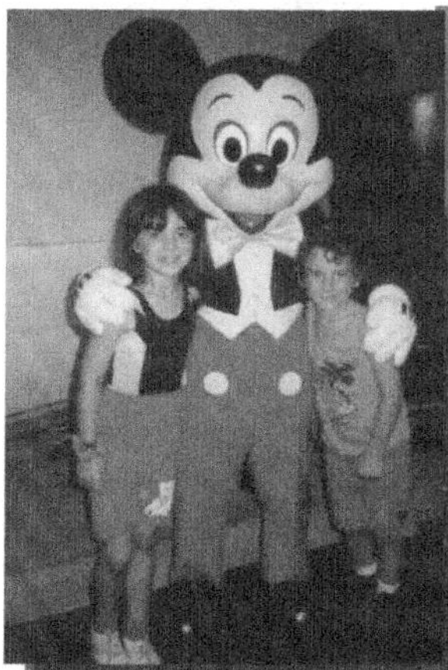
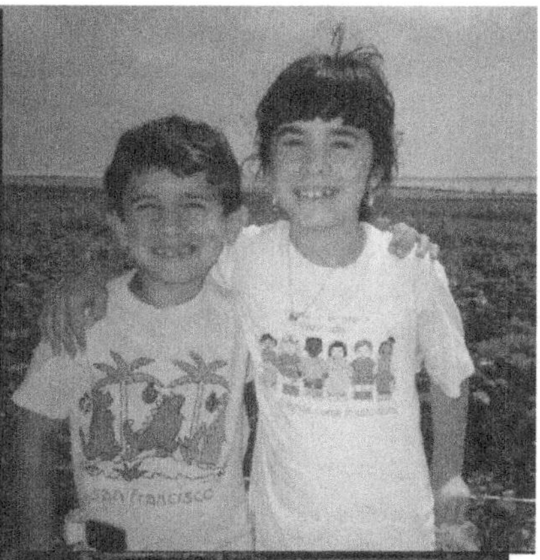
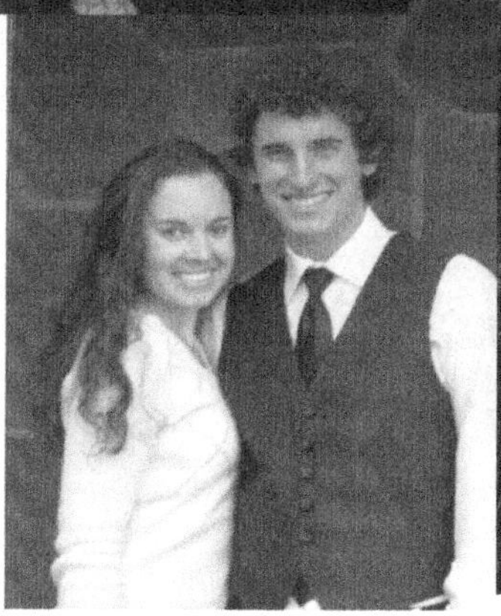
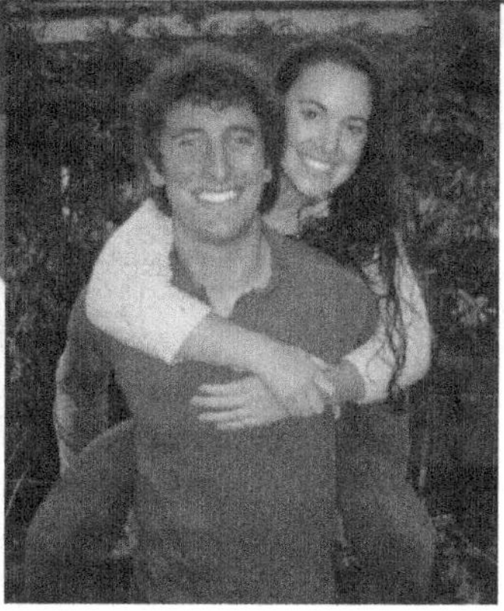

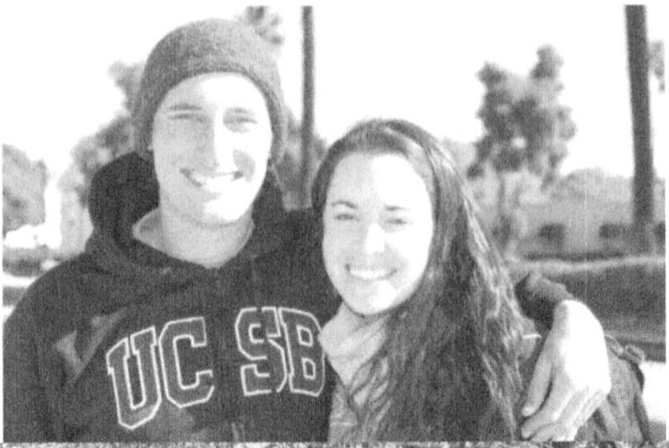
UC SB

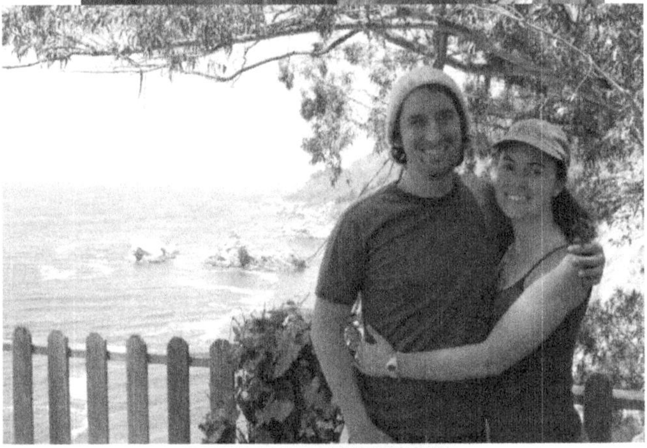

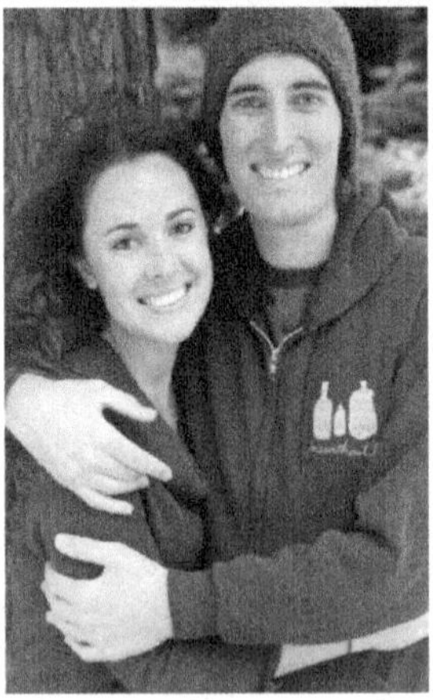

5
October's Song

Our daughter Alicia was born in October, the month Danny died, so this is the context of this reflection:

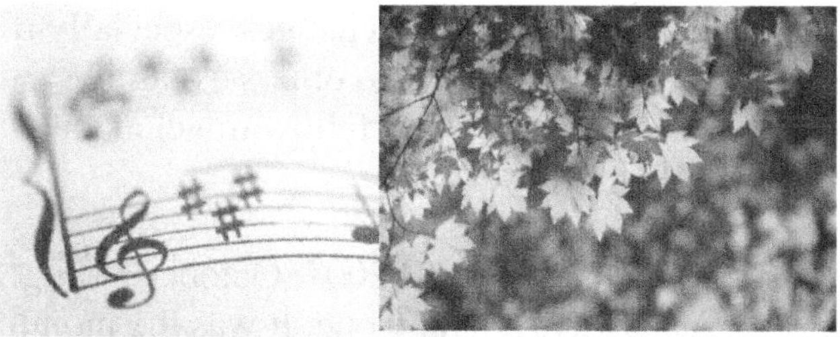

October sings of birth and death, the melodious happy sounds of recalling my daughter Alicia's birth on October 25, 1985 and the harsh discords of my son Danny's death on October 31, 2007. October's song is composed of the spectrum of life's emotions, the joy of the birth of a daughter, the pain and sadness of the death of a son. The lyrics of October's song reflect the changing colors of the season, the changing emotional moments of the cycle of life. The melodies are full of highs and lows, the soft chords that bring out the harmonies of life, and the sharps that touch the depth of life's losses.

October's song is not a solo. It needs a chorus made up of different voices: basses, tenors, sopranos, complimenting and supporting each other the way families, communities, celebrate our joys and hold us in our sorrows. Music transcends months, seasons, time but respects and reflects the changing moments life brings. A song is really never played or sung the same way twice because we are always confronting and rocked by life's changes, especially if we risk being close to others as family, parents, friends, and fellow travelers on life's journey.

Before October 31, 2007, October's song was always a happy one. It was the month we looked forward to our daughter's birthday: six, twelve, eighteen, twenty-one, and now twenty-three. I try to give her roses for each year of her life. She is really the flower of my life, blossoming now more than ever because the son I love so much, her beautiful brother, his mother's marvelous gift, is no longer with us, lost on October's last day. Danny sang, left his lyrics and music to brighten even the darkest October day, the day of his death. Danny's October song is unfinished, still being composed by those who loved him, learning to live without his smile, sense of humor, sensitivity, openness to others. The lyrics and melodies are being written as music's memory, drawing on remembering Danny, especially his songs, and the sounds Danny's spirit evokes in our hearts.

October's song is that of anyone who celebrates life: births, deaths, challenges in-between, seeking harmony in discords, clarity in confusion, hope in despair, light in darkness, open to the opportunities each new day brings. October's song is classical, rock, folk, rap, country, and spiritual, an evolving reflection of the music of life. October's song is the same and new each year, much as the colors of autumn are the same and different every October. October will always be happy and sad because of the celebration of life and death it brings, but October's song will always be filled with gifts given and received, discovered and yet to be found/shared, especially the joy of songs composed of life's lyrics and melodies.

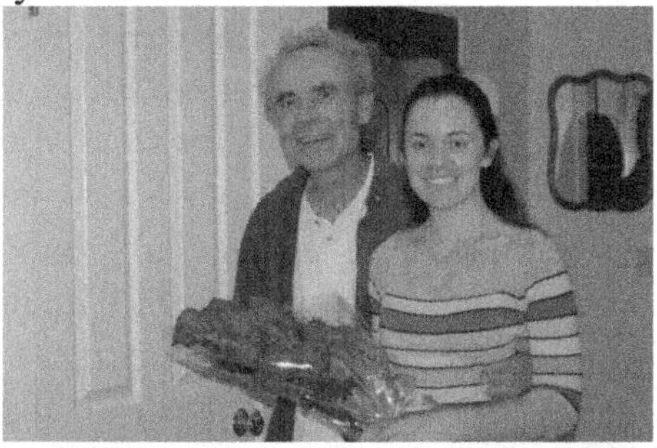

October 25, 2007, giving Alicia Rose 22 roses for her birthday.

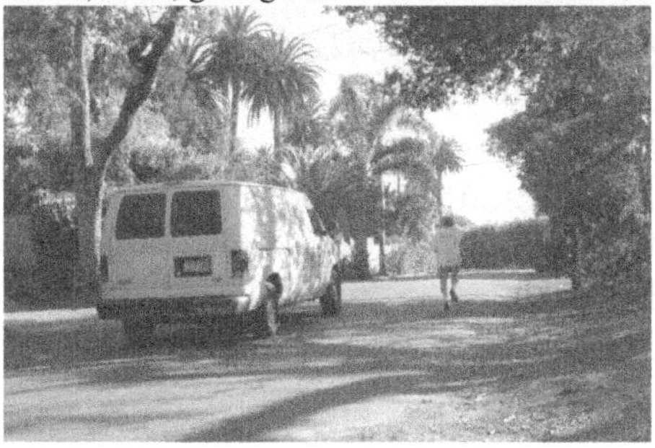

October 31, 2007, running by the van with Danny's body.

6
December

December is the month of Danny's birth. He was born on the twelfth day of the twelfth month at twelve minutes past twelve in the morning, so the number twelve was significant for him. He described himself in his autobiography, written for a project in his senior year of high school:

> My name is Daniel Joseph Riley. I am a leader in my high school, an ASB commissioner and active in several socially conscious clubs. I am a musician. I love to play guitar, drums, bass, piano, alto sax, and sing. I am a loving son, born and raised in California. I am an athlete of all sports, but primarily basketball and cross-country running. I am a student of history, language, love, and life. I am a poet and a politician. I am a brother and a boyfriend. I am a philosopher, friend, and comedian. I am a cousin to an enormous family of Irish Catholic heritage. I am the son of a teacher and the son of a priest. I am an optimist. Peace is always an answer. I am a movie-goer, and a sunset-watcher. I am a professional eater and mediocre chef. I am that really annoying kid in your AP Econ class with all the questions. I am white-skinned. I am a lover of learning. I am a lover of the question "why." I love mashed

> potatoes and banana pancakes. I love all types of good music. I am an experimentalist. I am a student of patience and modesty. I am a member of the human race. I love to wear sandals. I love to travel. I am semi-bilingual. I am middle-class. I am interested in the future. I am a brain cancer survivor.

The line that he is the "son of a priest" needs a little explanation. I was a Roman Catholic priest for fourteen years, but left the priesthood in 1983. Danny was born in 1987, and when he came to understand what it meant, he liked to share that his father was a priest. While I was not a parish priest and worked mostly in social ministries, I was called upon to be at the side of several children who died of cancer. I was struck by the strength of their parents in the face of such tragedy.

When Danny was diagnosed, I recalled those moments and wondered how I could bear such pain. Now I too have gone through the anguish of Danny's death and experienced the pain of missing him. Ironically, weakened by such a grave loss, I am discovering the strength of the human spirit, which I believe is touched by a deeper spiritual presence. It seems that this presence and the relationships that bind us are the source of that strength. Certainly Danny's strength guided me and still does. His strength will always be central to the story of my own life.

I tried to convey the gift of being his father in:

A Father's Reflection

On December 12, 1987, I stood by my new born son as he struggled for almost eight minutes to take his first breath. On October 31, 2007, I was by his side when he took his last. These two moments and the time in between spark some reflections which may touch the gift of a father's relationship to a child. I share them with a deep sense of gratitude for my son Danny and hope that all fathers will treasure whatever moments they have to be with their children.

Danny's life and death have helped me to appreciate my own life and not to fear the end of it. While Danny's almost twenty years were special for me, his last three were a testament to the depth of his spirit, love of those who touched his life in major or minor ways, and beacons of hope for all who must face life's harshest challenges.

On December 8, 2004, the doctor told Danny that he had a large tumor in the right front of his brain. This vibrant junior in high school, who was about to turn 17, took the news in stride and asked me: "How are you doing Poppy?" a phrase he would repeat many times over the next almost three years, along with: "Follow my lead." And how he led! He was a leader in smiling in adversity. His smile brought ones from older patients at the radiation clinic and Cancer centers, as well as the younger ones in the pediatric wards of the hospitals where his had three craniotomies and stays in between. Danny seemed to smile though cancer, which is true because he smiled throughout his short life.

Another theme of Danny's life was his love of music. As he would say: "music is my life." Through his music, spirit, and love of others, his life continues. His poetry also reflects his appreciation of others. One of his poems, given to me on my birthday in 2006, is a gift that any father would treasure, as I do:

From when I was young
You taught me to sing
Through tongue
Through heart
Through all of me.
I see now
That such a lesson
Is a gift of your spirit
Lacking any comparison
You lighten my burden
Of life and struggle,
Because of which, I know
you to care
Like no other individual

My wish is
that when I grow old
To carry with me
all that you've told
To resemble you
From all perspectives
And to have your heart
From which to love with.

Hear this when I say
That you are a blessing in my life
Every single day.

Love, Danny

"You lighten my burden of life and struggle..." A father helps a child face life's challenges, lighten the burden of these challenges by sharing them, loving the child through them, and affirming the relationship that develops along the way. My wish for all fathers is that they be a blessing in their children's lives every single day and that they always appreciate the blessings their sons and daughters are in theirs.

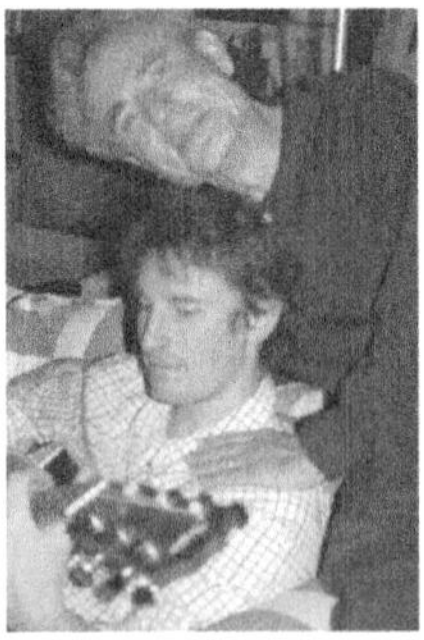

7
The Basketball Backboard

Danny's story is very personal but I have a sense that others might benefit from these reflections, which is why I am weaving them together. Also, this project helps me move on without leaving Danny behind. Here is another reflection about the happy times we spent competing at basketball in our driveway:

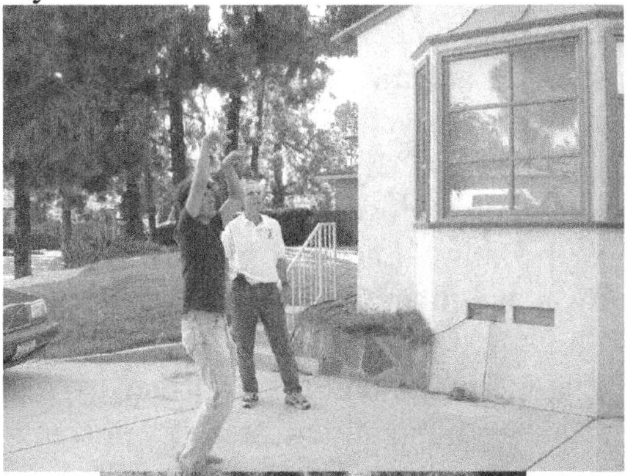

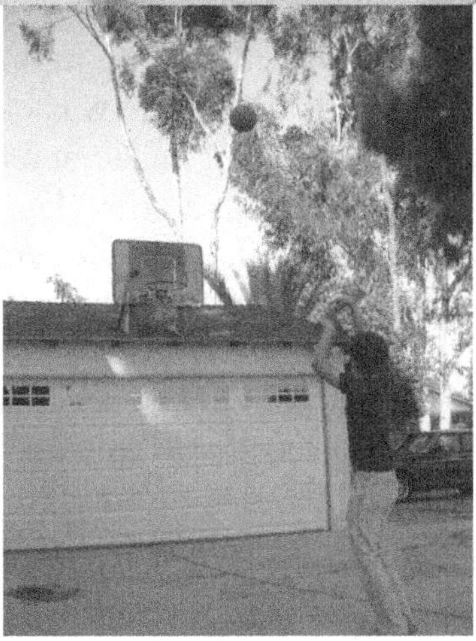

The plastic backboard was cracked and the wood that was holding it up was rotting, so the symbol of happy times playing basketball needed to come down. Yet, I was reluctant to do so and cried when I did because Danny was the one who used it the most and put up the best shots. It drew Danny and me together, competing for the unheralded honors that usually remained our secret. I actually beat him once in a great while and loved to razz him about it, which usually sparked a "no mercy" game that I lost badly. However, when I spent any time with Danny, I never lost; I always came away a winner.

Playing basketball in our driveway was Danny's main athletic activity during his treatments his junior and senior years of high school. Making a long jump shot seemed to validate that he was okay, strong, and healing. Playing music and basketball were two markers of a good day, despite the pressures of school, the treatments, and the underlying questions his illness posed. They were gifts he could develop and share, and I was the main recipient of his basketball skills. As hard as it was to take down the symbol of that sharing, it was time because Danny shares in different ways now, ones that are emerging as I listen to my heart, see those who loved him honoring him by smiling again, living his mantra of seeking Love, Life, and Light in their lives and sharing these gifts.

No more three-pointers in our driveway, but plenty of memories of the ones Danny made and hopes that his spirit of play and fun surprise me in the days ahead.

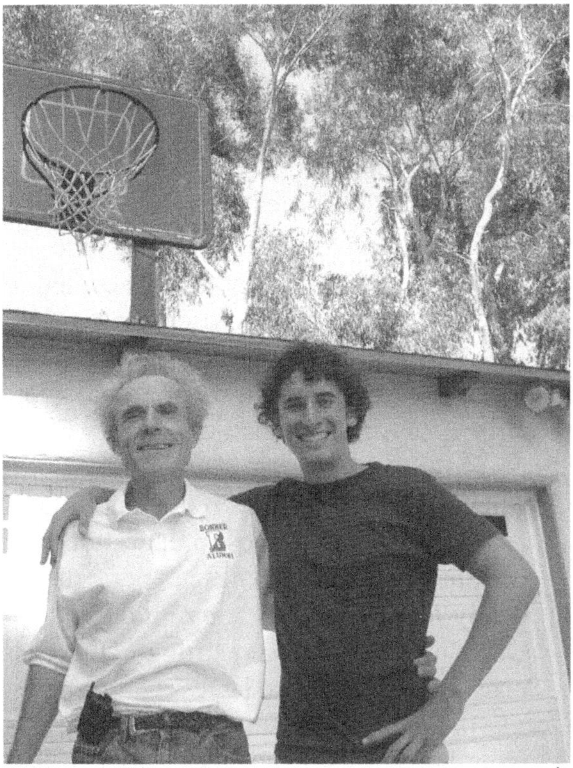

8
Danny's Values/Poems

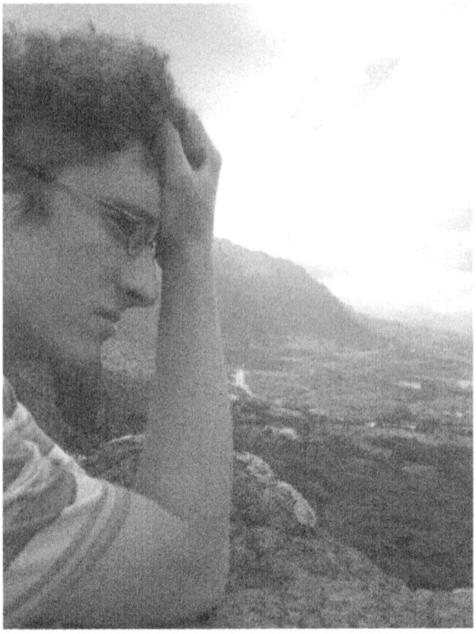

Many have commented that Danny was wise beyond his years and that his maturity seemed to strengthen him and drew him closer to others in the midst of his life-threatening challenge. In a reflection on leaving high school, he wrote about how bad times helped him mature:

> Then of course there were the bad times. In a way, I gained the most preparation for and insight into life from these experiences. One of my favorite quotes is by Frederick Douglas, 'If there is no struggle, there is no progress.' This quote states what I mean to say in a very beautiful way. Through all the pain, late nights, headaches, blood, tears,

> and cancer, I have matured faster than I ever thought possible. I believe this to be one of my greatest strengths as I prepare for college-life and beyond. I feel that I have matured enough as a person to understand the significance of my education, the significance of my friends and family, and the significance of living a full, well-rounded life. I feel mature enough to take college life seriously, and in a manner that will further my growth as a human being. I feel mature enough to know when to laugh, when to cry, when to fight, and when to make peace. These are some of the things that I have learned that I know I will carry with me for the rest of my life.

Danny carried this maturity through the rest of his short life and it was one of the qualities that helped him achieve his goal to live a normal life, despite brain cancer. Danny's life reflected an inner strength that shaped that way he communicated with others and faced the good and bad times of his life.

Danny was baptized a Catholic and often went to Sunday Mass with me, but his own beliefs shaped his life. Perhaps that is why he was so strong in the face of such challenges. He wrote about his beliefs and values (these are presented just as they were written on this laptop):

Dear God

and im going to seek out your advice. im going to seek out your wisdom. i dont know who you are. i dont know how you exist. but you are everything that is in all of me and all of us. please forgive me for not acknowledging it sooner. but ive been in such a haze my entire life. just give me the strength to admit im wrong. give me the compassion to start anew. give me the happiness to love. you are nature. you are so much more than me. i want to be part of you. i want to experience you through love and charity and laughter and happiness. so when i am lost and when i am confused and when i am sad, i will come back to you, nature, god, love, soul, world, color, sky, wind, earth. and admit that you are more than i. and that i need you in my life. i will accept everything. a servant to all. a student of all.

World of Love

Make me into a world of love
Passion in my soul and kindness in my heart
Bend the skin which binds my cast
Heal me once and it will forever last.
Take me from the devil's rays
Hold me close for all my days
The sky is bright with tender hope
I feel it in the words ive wrote.

Simply am I on a path
Alone and blind I search and laugh
To find my peace that is my quest
To fulfill my life is my end at last.

Instrument of Thy Love

Its something like a destiny
I for you and you for me.

The strength that lies in three thin lines
The shared presence within two minds

Make me an instrument of thy love
To bless and keep these bonds we hold.

A Prayer

ill say a prayer from the past
and for the future
waking up to the morning light
ill think of you and remember why
i said a prayer on this day
just so i could hear you say

dont you know me?
dont you know me by now?

i spoke of all my hopes and dreams
so feather light and full of cream
so tender young and full of tears
could it surpass the years?
that ive spent my mind and

forgotten this heart
that you hinted at.
i wish i could get it back.

dont you know me?
dont you know me by now?

someday we'll see.
someday we'll see.
dont forget about me.
dont forget about me.

Desire

so when i say that i need something it is half true. i dont need the object itself. but rather the desire for the object. this is how life should be lived. like those people who see the glass half full. they do not see what they lack, they see what they have to gain. they see what they desire. this desire fuels their being and existence. it makes everything worth while. so whenever you have doubt or whenever you feel pain, think of all that there is to gain. because he who lacks everything has everything to strive for. the poorest among us have the most desire. and desire is the essence of life. always be aware of what you want.

Give Back

at times, all i want is to give back. not with purpose. not with agenda. drown out the glory in it. just to be. be something real. be alive. be love. there is nothing else i would ask for. i take in all that i give out. and all i give is love. seemless and simple. oh please dont say this is fake. pray my vision never break. love and live. laugh and cry. tears are nothing more than fear falling from your face. such a hidden grace, as can be seen in these eyes. and all of our eyes. open your eyes.

Passing

and you lift
passing,
beyond your comforts and homes.
leaving all your loves and mundane charms.

and you soar
passing,
above those colored specks
that coat the ground and crane your neck.

and you dream
passing,
through your faults and dreary traits
exploding from them wearing ribbons and bows.
if there ever was

a time
when this was easy
id like to live it.

Harmony

lost in size and lift in your chest. digest these means of feeling alive. with wide eyes and fevered sighs. shaking tears of joy. gone from sight but closer to heart. a type of love which does not depart. a world of solutions to its own problems. one mind of matter used to solve them. like an essay, answerless. morals dont apply. but used to memorize. the pricks and sparks that singe skin. a way that leaves you dreaming in. dreaming in towards me. such is harmony.

Youth

and maybe we are all just in this haze that is youth. blinded by our love and ideals. i cant tell. when im older will i laugh at all these words that ive saved up? will i say that i was naive? that i was a fool to love so deeply? if there is one thing that i can keep with me, through my entire life, it would be my love. i dont want to fade away. i dont want to become cold. i always want to love everything just as passionatly as i do now. i dont fear pain. ill accept it. embrace it even. just let me keep my love.

Sharing Life

a moment is nothing, if it is not shared. qualitiy of life will be qualified on how much time you spend with the ones you love.
everything else is meaningless.
im convinced that there is no difference in our experiences. there is no way that someone's life can be harder or easier than anyone else's. because we all see our own lives in such a drama that everything has a great amont of significance. we all go through the same amount of pain and struggle.

Ivory Angel

im tired of all the killing
why cant we care for the poor?
with so much hatred and anger
we all can do a little more.
come and kiss them ivory angel
they need to see your healing light
come and kiss them ivory angel
the last thing we need is another fight
with all of us
bound together with our hearts
we can find the answers
to the questions that keep us apart.

Be Humble

Be humble. the biggest mistake you can
make is thinking that you understand it all.
because you dont. and you wont. always try
and learn something new. always take
everyone's advice. always doubt yourself!
no one likes someone who seems godly and
perfect. we want something real. we dont
want to be compared. we want to be equals.
i want to be your equal. or less than.
be humble to the world and the world will
be humble to you.
be humble to God and God will be humble
to you.
treat everything else as you would want it
reflected upon yourself. because everything
is reflected back upon yourself.
modesty.

Selfless

to be selfless and care more about someone
else than you do for yourself is the closest
we can be to having a divine trait. it is the
closest to imitating god as we can ever be.
as humans we are built to be selfish and only
care about our own well being. when we
manage to care about others more than we
do ourselves then we have truly reached a
state of enlightened existence, surpassing all
boundaries of our human form.
in life, i dont think that there is a difference

between pain and joy. it is definitly possible for someone to experience pure joy without pain, invariably. you dont need the contrast of experiencing pain in order to experience joy, because the emotions are one and the same. it is just a different reflection of the same emotion.

Being Alone

From being alone i have learned many things. i have learned how to deal with sorrow and how to deal with happiness. When alone, you become more thoughtful. from this you become more in tune with your true self. a more harmonious person so to speak.
As a person who has attained true self awareness or true harmony with oneself, you seem "cool" to the outside world. calm and collected. attractive and envied.
Needing nothing but internal peace to obtain your happiness, you seem to have a better grasp on life than others around you. they see this and try to get closer to you, in order to understand the source of your peace of mind.
That source is your constant internal probing. thoughtfulness. acceptance to being alone.

Love

When the pesimists say that love doesnt last, I have to disagree. It seems to me that they have never known the true meaning of love. Love isnt purly lust and passion between two people, it is the utmost friendship. I agree that lust does not maintain at the same level at all times. However friendship doesnt fade away on its own. Because of this, love does not fade with time. When quoting an example of a failed love over time, it just proves that they were never in love in the first place. Friendship is the key.

Care For

what can i do with these curved lines?
what can we feel in this short time?
actually, i dont believe in what i dont care for
and i dont care for time or hate or unhappiness.

all of these different dramas are so intertwined
we may not see it at all but if we only stand tall
peer above the horizon line, see the drop and sphere.

i dont know why we even try sometimes.

everything youve ever done
ever choice youve ever made
in interest of your fortune
and avoidance. youre so afraid.

and its my choice to take a step back and
observe,
the dismal haze and sterile ways
in which we go about our lives.

i dont know why we even try sometimes.

and then im reminded of why i care
and what i care for
by the slightest twist on the handle
of that red crusted door.

it holds back all my lust and pain
but rather breathes life to my true desire
where some would find it unpleasing to
explain
that floating feeling it sets afire.

but whatever presents itself,
im glad to be here with all of you.
so glad to be here with all of you.
in our mutual ignorance.

remember. we only think about ourselves.
watch me break that.

i choose not to drown out my doubt and fear
but rather stare them down. break them with

my mind.
the bottle never had style. only blind guiding guile.

True Self

In order to be my true self
spend time on myself
meditate,
breathe,
sing,
write,
listen,
be.
Be conscious of my environment
And how it influences me.

Be conscious of the fog of chemo
And how it affects my mental clarity.

Fight back against these influences, which mischaracterize my true self.

The Sun

the sun is my lover
holding me close with its warm touch
but sometimes its nails do cut in
and the heat is too much
i just need to cool down
and find me some quiet space
at my friend the winds house
cool air always inhabits his place

but eventually i always break
and come running back to my solar love
she commands the sky and earth above
there's nothing more beautiful than her
setting rays
reflecting off the passing clouds
blown by my good friend the wind
when she is gone i have nothing left
the air is far too cold for me to smile.
wind cannot comfort me the way she does
i miss her most when the rain comes.

Love Everyone

i would rather love everyone, than hate those
who are different.

All of me

it will be awhile before you notice all of me.

Alone

when something amazing happens to you
but no one is with you to experience it.

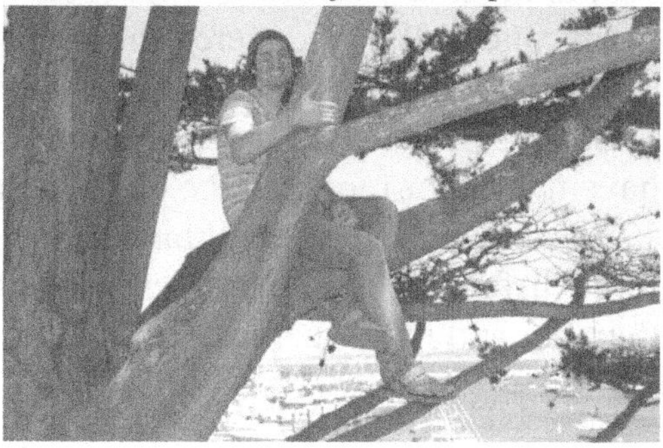

9
Letters/Answers

In this computer age, letters are a lost art replaced by e-mails and text messages. However, Danny wrote some to show his appreciation for the gifts he received. He also had to provide answers on applications for scholarships. Like his poems, they bring out his maturity and focus, despite his challenges:

Dear Donor,

I would like to personally thank you for your generous donation to the American Cancer Society. As a student at University of California Santa Barbara, your contribution has helped me in many ways. Your donation has allowed me to put more focus into the issues that affect my daily life, such as chemo and school, without having to constantly worry about how I'm going to pay for it all.

As of several days ago, I celebrated my two year anniversary of being diagnosed with brain cancer. We discovered the tumor after a weekend of terrible headaches and one fateful CAT-SCAN. I had a craniotomy to have the tumor removed the day after my 17th birthday. Since then, I have undergone three different chemotherapies, radiation therapy, and radio (gamma knife) surgery

At first my tumor spread to the side of my brain, and I actually had a scan a month ago where both tumors decreased in size. As of my last MRI scan, both of them appear to be stable.

At UCSB, I am a freshman English major, but I am pretty confident that I am going to change me major to something like political science or philosophy. Right now I am taking courses in Philosophy, Religious Studies, and Art History. However, my main interest is music. Unfortunately, I won't be able to enter into a music major program because they no longer offer a guitar emphasis, which I would prefer. I've been playing guitar for 3 years now and I love to write songs and improvise. I listen to an expansive collection of music from jazz, to folk, to rock, to hip-hop. My dream is to become an accomplished guitar player, for my own sake, not to be famous or rich, but just to develop my abilities to the fullest so that I may enjoy my life through my guitar and music. Your donation has allowed me to strive for my goals of living life to the fullest and using education as a means of evolving and progressing myself as an individual.

> Once again I would wish you to know how much your donation has meant to my life personally, and all the other students like me who benefit from the American Cancer Society. From the bottom of my heart, thank you very much for your kindness, generosity, and compassion. It will not be forgotten.
>
> Truly,
>
> Daniel J Riley

In his application for a Pediatric Brain Tumor Foundation scholarship, Danny answered several questions including:

> **Describe what you consider the single most important project or activity in which you have participated that has benefited your community.**
>
> The single most important project, which I have been involved in, is the SHADES project. This project is aimed to raise awareness and discussion regarding racial prejudice. The acronym refers to "Simply Honoring All Diverse Ethnicities." I was introduced and invited to participate in this program's student panel. In the program we view several film clips confronting racial discrimination. After each clip, the panel discusses it based on their own ethnic

perspective. Two moderators help facilitate the discussion for a large student and adult audience. We will be putting on this program for the mayor of San Diego and councilmen in the near future. I feel I have made a significant contribution as a leader within my school and community by being willing to address difficult questions of race and prejudice in an open and thoughtful manner.

Why is going to college important to you and what are your future plans?

Going to college is very important to me because education is the best way for me to grow and become a better person. I have always dreamed of going to college, and using the experience to better myself and the world around me. One of the greatest aspects of college, which I have looked forward to for many years, is being able to choose my own field of study. This is appealing to me because I enjoy learning for learning's sake. In the classroom, I am that somewhat annoying student who is always asking too many questions, and always craving more knowledge. But the main reason why I wish to go to college is for the overall experience: meeting new people, living on my own, playing college sports, taking unique classes, etc. I can't wait to experience the college atmosphere, and make the most of it.

I have not yet decided upon any precise career goals, but at the moment I am very much interested in English, political science, and philosophy. I hope to begin my studies in one of these fields. A consistent goal of mine is to become a better writer. I am fascinated by the power of the English language and wish to further develop my ability to use it, in all forms, from poetry to argumentative essays. Political science is in my blood, passed down to me from my baby boom parents. I have grown up in a very politically conscious home, and for this I am so grateful. I would love to continue my education in political science so to empower me to change the world. Philosophy is another passion of mine. Awareness of the world around me challenges me to grow as an individual being. My love of philosophy is fueled by eagerness to learn about life. For me, this is the most fascinating subject. I am also an avid musician and will always be devoted to that part of my life. My dream would be to find a career that encouraged and inspired the continuation of my music.

If you had to state a theme or moral to your life story, what would it be?

Life is meant to love.

What words would you share with a newly diagnosed brain tumor patient?

Smile. This will be the best thing that has ever happened to you. Enjoy it. What is there to be afraid of? Feel the cancer in you, and beat it with love.

Danny smiled through his journey with cancer even before and after his three brain surgeries:

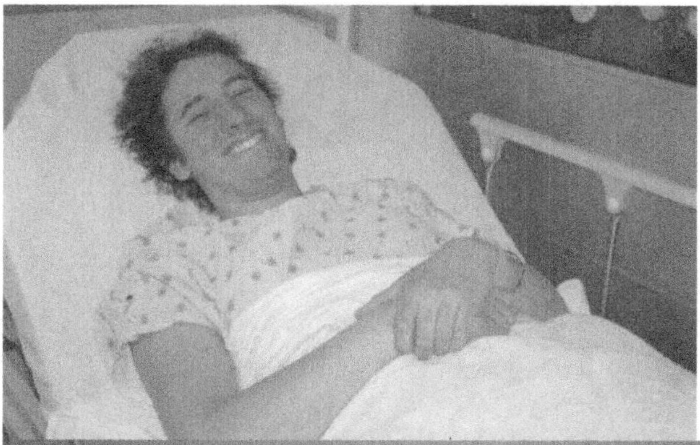

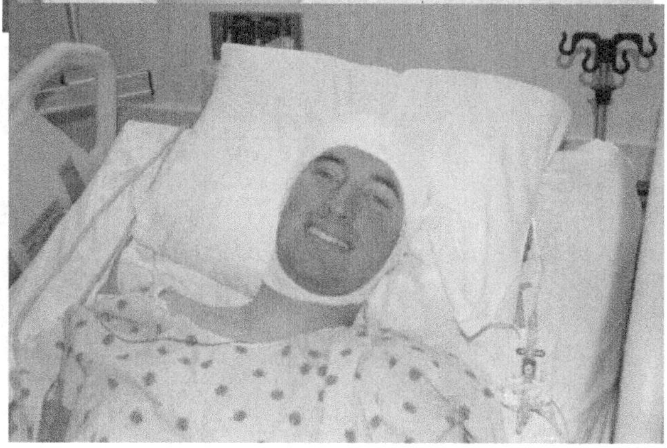

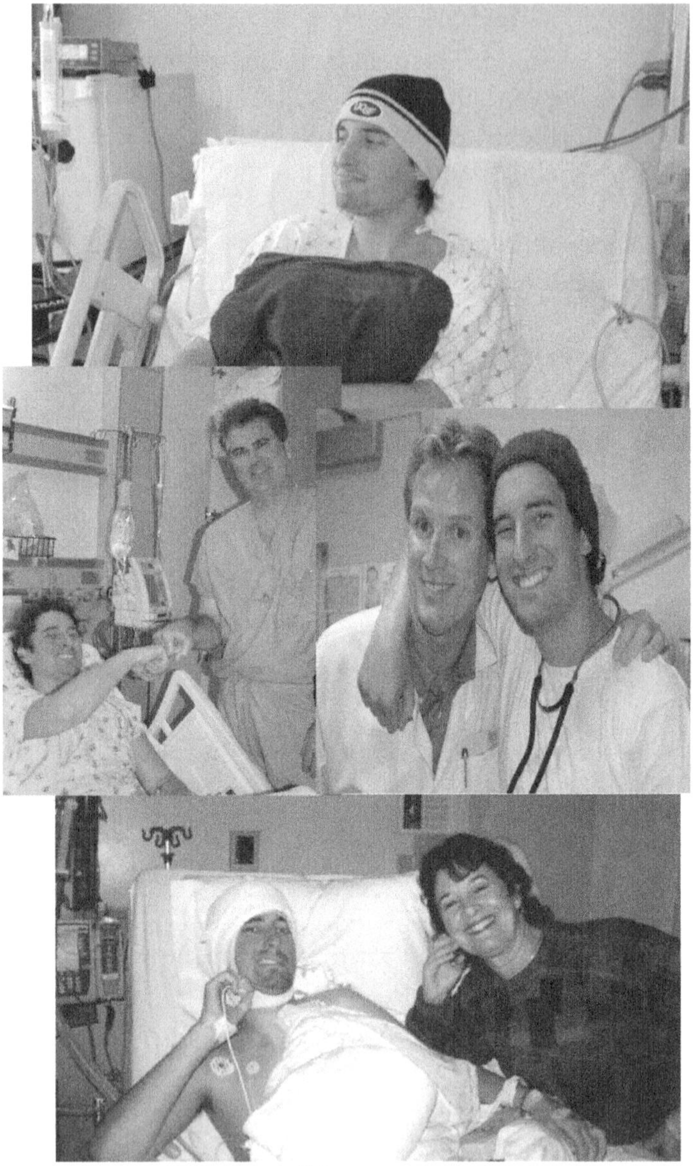

10
Love/Life/Light

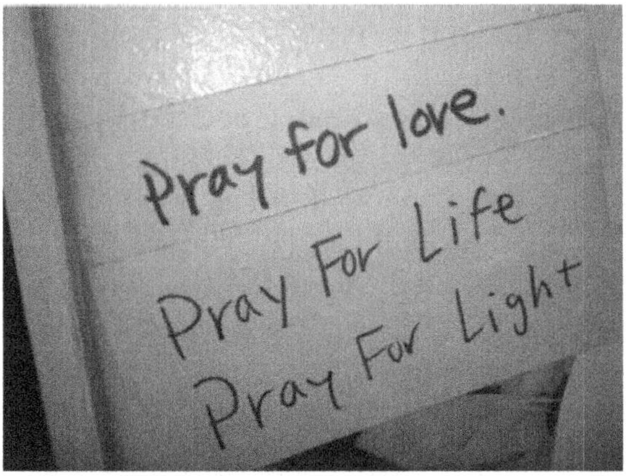

On the wall in Danny's room

If Danny had a mantra or theme that colored his story, it would be: "love, life, light." When small groups gathered around his bed to pray with him, this would be his way of concluding the prayers and being sure they would end on an up-beat note. These three words seemed to be Danny's consistent message to all of those who shared his journey, his focus that enabled him not only to accept the challenges of each day, but embrace them with deep appreciation for all those who helped him along the way.

In March of 2006, in the middle of his freshman year at UCSB, the tumor progressed to such a degree that he needed a second craniotomy, which we had performed by the skilled team at UCSF Medical Center. Maggi and I drove to Santa

Barbara to pick Danny up to drive to San Francisco for the surgery. It was surreal! The campus was buzzing, young men and women biking to classes, fooling around in the dorms, or laying on the lawn under the warm California sun. Yet, we were there to give our son a ride to San Francisco for his second brain surgery in less than two years. Danny was optimistic, even jovial. As he was leaving his dorm, some of his buddies gave him hugs and on leaving Danny yelled: “Give me a call! If I answer, I survived, if I don’t, I’m dead.” Danny survived another complicated surgery which did not cure him, but gave hope for longer survival and further treatment. When he left the hospital, Danny wrote these words in an e-mail he sent on April 17, 2007:

> Thank you to everyone who gave up some of their time to pay me a visit or send an email, card, or phone call, thought, or prayer. None of them went without being truly appreciated. i am so blessed to have such great family and friends to support me throughout all of these times. I honestly would not want my life to be played out any other way than it currently has, because i could not imagine it without any greater presence of Love, Life, or Light than it currently has.

A week or so later, we drove south and dropped him off at UCSB, where he resumed his studies, camaraderie with his friends, writing poetry, and songs about love, life, and light. Thanks to the assistance of the University's Program for Students with Disabilities, ongoing care from the Student Health Center, the Cancer Center of Santa Barbara, and Kaiser in Los Angeles, as well the help of his cousins in Santa Barbara and close friends like Catherine and Mike, Danny completed his freshman year with honors.

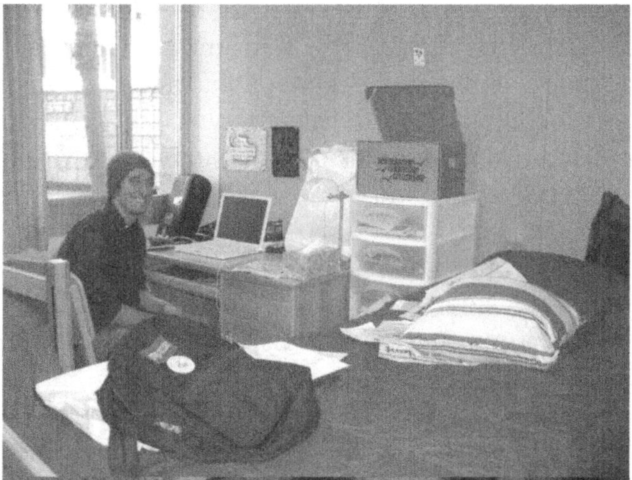

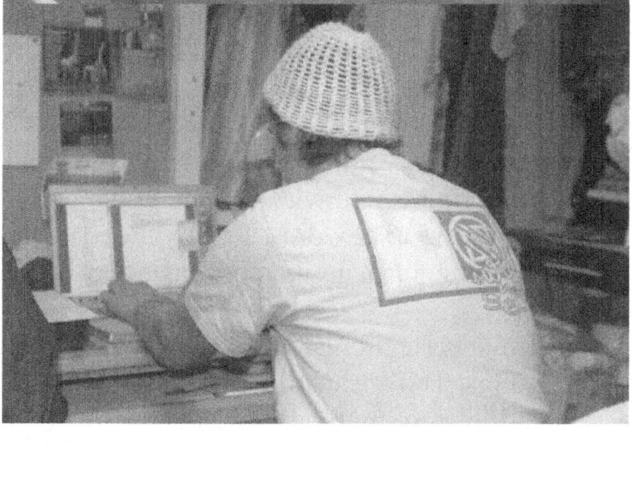

11
Music

As Danny wrote, his dream was "…to become an accomplished guitar player, for my own sake, not to be famous or rich, but just to develop my abilities to the fullest so that I may enjoy my life through my guitar and music." Anyone who has listened to his music knows that he was well on his way to realizing his dream. Even in his most difficult days he enjoyed playing his guitar and singing his songs for others to appreciate and enjoy. Danny described music as "one of my dearest passions." and wrote about his love of music:

> From a young age I have been drawn toward music in a very soulful way. Just the hum of a guitar string or whisper of a melody can send chills down my spine. I love it. In fact, if you count humming and singing at the kitchen table while crunching on cheerios, I've been making music since I was about five. Besides humming and singing, I now play piano, alto saxophone, guitar, bass, and drums. In recent years I have become increasingly interested in songwriting and performing solo with just my guitar and voice. In other words, I enjoy the idea of creating music in its most basic form.
>
> I'm a perfectionist when it comes to my own songs. This makes for an ever-present struggle to improve the quality of my music.

My biggest frustration comes from writing lyrics. I am often dissatisfied with the tone and meaning of the lyrics I compose. This is one reason why I wish to become a better writer. To develop my writing abilities further, I want to study English or possibly creative writing.

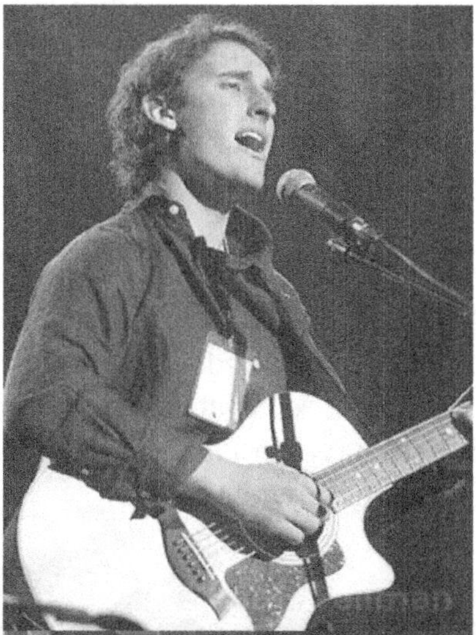

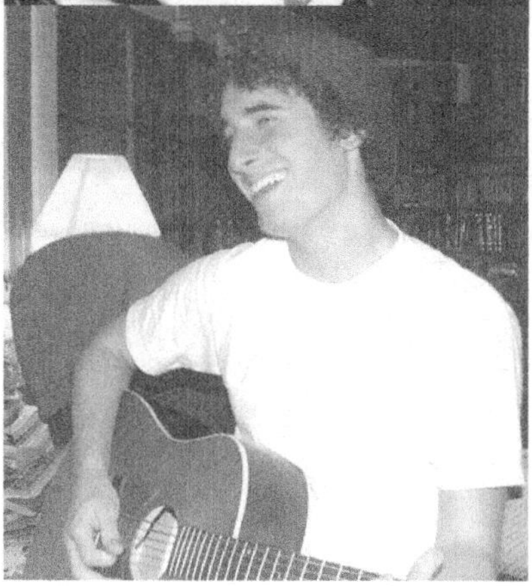

Danny had some help in his guitar playing from his cousin Kim's boyfriend and later husband, Jack Johnson, who not only helped with the guitar but with all aspects of his life. On December 12, 2004, Danny's 17th birthday and the day before his first brain surgery, Jack drove down from Los Angeles, where he was working on the music for the film "Curious George" to our home in Chula Vista, just south of San Diego. Jack's visit really helped Danny, especially when he shared that he had to have brain surgery due to a serious accident surfing he had in Hawaii when he was the same age as Danny.

Jack and Danny also played some of Jack's songs, delighting Danny's friends. As I listened and watched, I wondered what effect the next day's surgery would have on Danny's ability to sing and play the songs he loved.

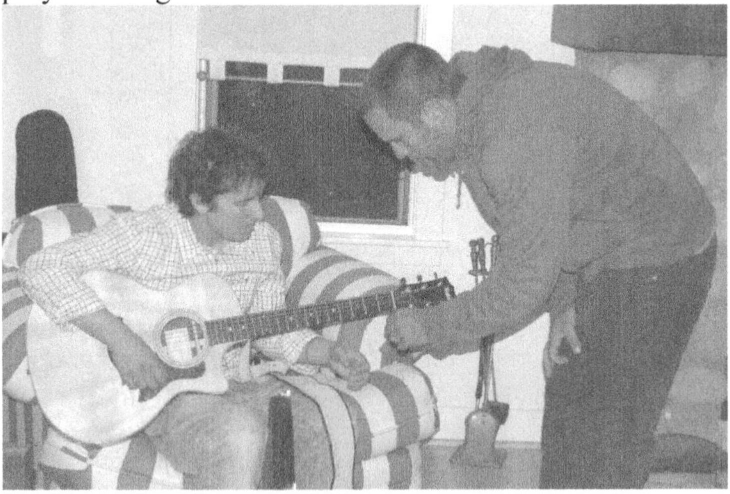

Jack giving Danny some tips.

Danny used music to express his hopes and joys as well as his fears and sorrows, sometimes juxtaposed in the same song. One of Danny's songs "Silent Cry" was written shortly after the Tsunami of December 2004 and his pathology report which occurred within a day of it. It tells of pain but speaks of hope, which symbolized Danny's life.

Silent Cry

I can't believe my eyes
I can't believe my ears
the ground has shook
the waves have crashed.
All those innocent lives don't deserve the grief
they cover their eyes and trust in their belief
the moment is frozen by the silent cry
and inaudible scream tell me why

How does one survive such pain, such pain?
how do others live with such shame, such shame?
how does one dream if there's no hope?
how does one sing as they choke?

Oh pray wise man let your charm burn into the twilight
watch as the smoke rolls out with the tide
and hovers above the sea
the spirts will rise up from the red sand and take you old man by the hand

guide you through this tragedy.
How does one survive such pain such pain?
how do others live with such shame such shame?
how does one dream if there's no hope?
how does one sing as they choke?

If I could only mend a heart
or give something back for them to start
we are all the same anyway
we all need love in the simplist of ways.

There's deeper magic at work here,
don't be afraid.

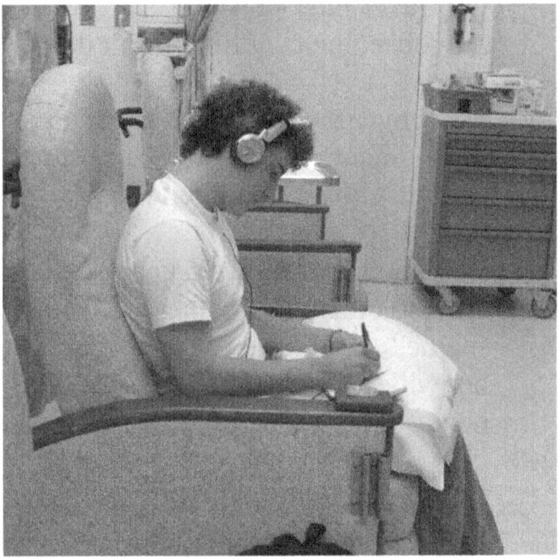

Music was Danny's companion during treatments.

One of Danny's poems shows the power of a song:

> When you don't know what you are writing
> for
> It is life
> Spun together and thrown into the cosmic
> world
> And all you have is time to burn.
> And it does
> In red pages of ancient lines
> And simple stories to pass the time.
> Hear the shaking pierce of lacking purpose
> It radiates from this population
> Stripping skies of their eternal glow.
> words are only an excuse to do nothing
> being my next point
> in this essay on living slowly and breathing
> lightly.
> it is only when these words are given a voice
> a purpose, through song, becomes their
> name
> this is what you are writing for.

While Danny was serious about his love of music, everything was open to humor. Danny and I had our own way of joking with each other, one of which was to leave prank messages on voicemail. Danny extended this to others as well, including his godfather Joe Dibos, who is a lawyer. Danny would call Joe pretending he was a judge and make up some mischief.

My prank messages were blander but once in a while I would get a good one, as with the call from Johnny One Note. The context was that Danny was a frequent purchaser of songs from iTunes, the ones you download for $.99 each. What began as a few songs gradually grew due to Danny's love of every type of music and my reluctance to refuse to pay for this expensive habit. Thus the phony message that "came" from iTunes. I called to inform him that he was the best customer we had, downloading numerous songs at great expense, which must reflect a very generous father. Identifying myself as Johnny One Note, and disguising my voice, I congratulated him on his extensive taste in music and encouraged him to keep the downloads coming and to thank his father for his generous support. Danny got a kick out of it and it became a standing joke that Johnny One Note called to say keep the songs rolling.

Most humor has a kernel of truth to it. For this prank, it was Danny's love of all types of music. Through iTunes and other means, he gathered a wide variety of music, which he enjoyed talking about and sharing. Music was not only his passion but a source of inspiration, healing, and wholeness. Whether it was listening, playing or singing a song, Danny was most alive in that moment. I and others who were there will never forget several of those magic moments: In January of 2005, Danny was asked to play for the morning service at the United Church of Christ in Carlsbad, where his grandfather was pastor emeritus. Danny chose to play Ben

Harper's song "Waiting on An Angel," a beautiful ballad that was even more poignant when Danny performed it. Danny touched the strings and hit every note and in so doing seemed to proclaim that he was healing and happy, a gift shared with a welcoming community who all knew his story.

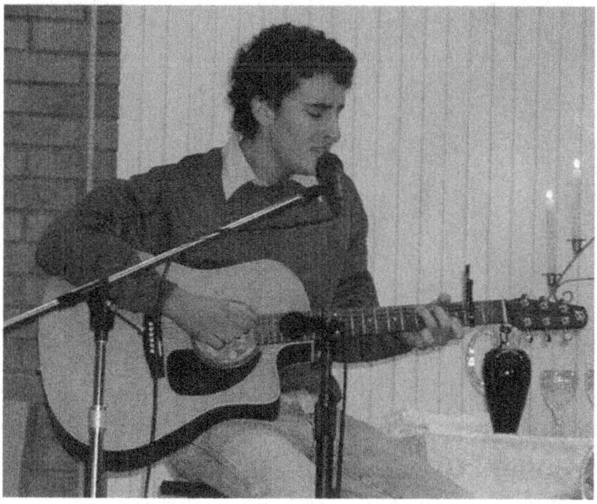

In March of 2007, Danny sang his signature song "Through Their Eyes" during the Solutions for Dreamers Benefit Concert for Heal the Ocean in Santa Barbara. A few days earlier he had an infusion of two strong chemotherapy drugs and he was still feeling the debilitating effects just before he was to perform. Yet, when Matt MacAvene announced that Danny Riley was going to sing during his set and he came on the stage, he was fully there. When he finished, the over 2,000 people thanked him with a standing ovation.

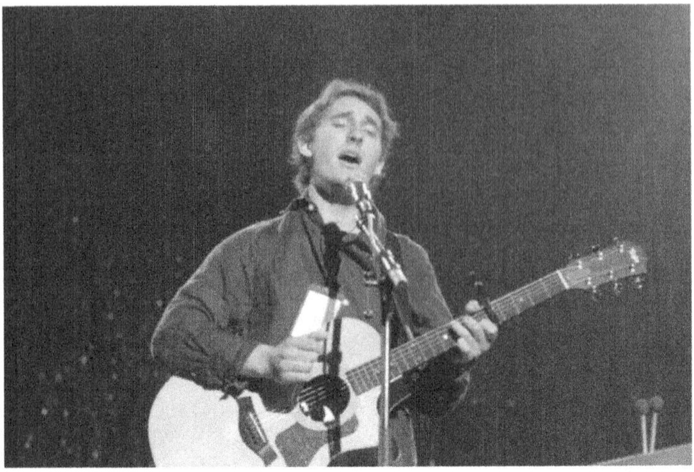

In July of 2007 the nausea and pain were consuming Danny, limiting his abilities, especially to play and sing. However, he was determined to learn Leonard Cohen's famous song Hallelujah, so he could play it in August for a celebration honoring his Grandpa. Despite his weakness, he learned it and could play it beautifully. However, as the nausea and pain increased he would have to go to the Cancer Center of San Diego for pain management and hydration, One evening after a day at the Cancer Center, we came home to Maggi's loving greeting and a surprise visit from his girlfriend Catherine and her mother Elvie, who brought arroz pollo, which she prepared for Danny. Revived by the time at the Cancer Center, the good company and food, Danny obliged us by playing Hallelujah, with Elvie holding up a page with the lyrics that he had forgotten. Only four of us

witnessed it, but we thought he would play for others in August.
Unfortunately, August brought more nausea and pain and his third brain surgery so he did not get to play Hallelujah at the August event. However, we did record Danny's singing it on September 21 at Jack Johnson's studio in Los Angeles, where we stopped on our way to UC Santa Barbara. Danny was really weak and his singing reflected this, but he got through it, even soaring on the line about standing "...before the Lord of Song." This song and others Danny loved show his appreciation of music as a healer for broken bodies and a broken world.

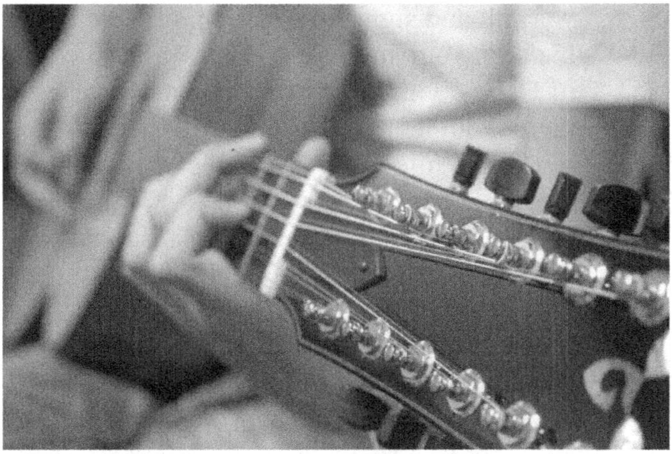

Danny trying out a twelve-string guitar

12
Touch

The story of Danny is about the way he touched people, which I tried to show in the following reflection and accompanying pictures:

Hand on My Shoulder

Danny's memory is of a vibrant, caring boy who, as he hit seventeen, had to face brain cancer, live with it, and die at age 19 as a result of it. Central to remembering Danny is recalling the way he touched others with his warmth and signs of affection, especially his hand on your shoulder. Picture after picture of Danny with others show his arm over their shoulders as if to pull them gently into his life. While Danny's hand cannot be over my shoulder anymore, I still feel it pulling me gently into his new life, gesturing to me that his is still part of mine. I share this in the hope that family and friends who had Danny's hand on their shoulders will have the same feeling, a sense of Danny Boy still traveling with them, sharing his journey into never-ending Love, Life, and Light.

The pictures that follow are just a sample but are a vivid recollection of Danny embracing those who touched his life and allowed him to touch theirs with his genuine expressions of affection. Danny's hand on your shoulder was never forced because he really cared about others and reached out to show that. Danny's hand on your shoulder and his smile were gifts he seemed to want to share to help you feel good, despite the challenges you knew he was facing.

As we experience life's mysteries and wonder, may Danny's gentle touch be a part of that journey, gesturing us to seek the gifts he loved: music, family, friends, and the smiles sharing these gifts bring.

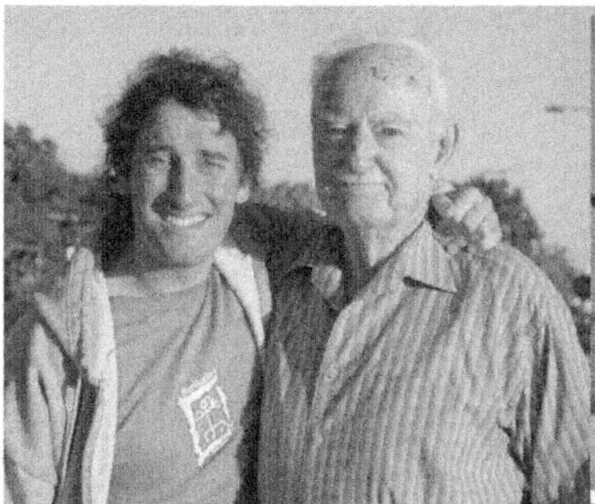

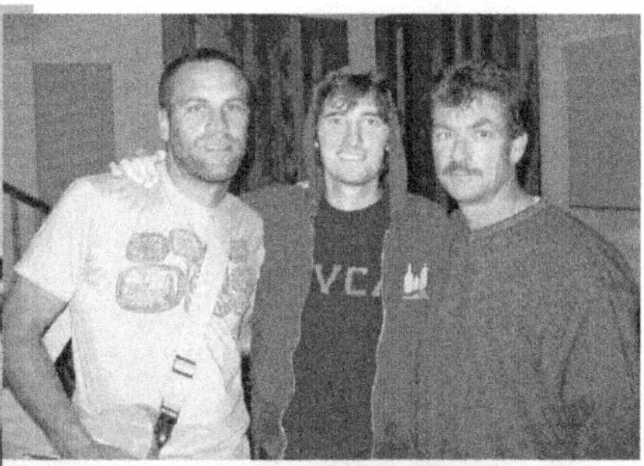

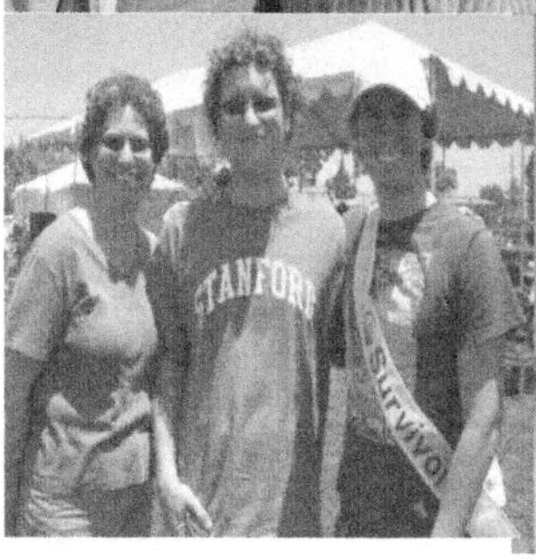

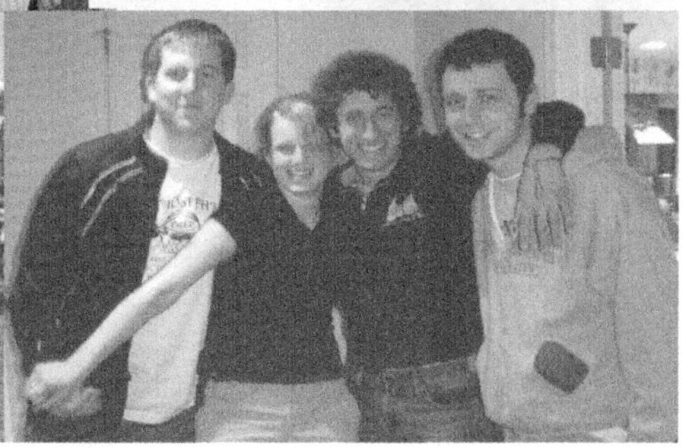

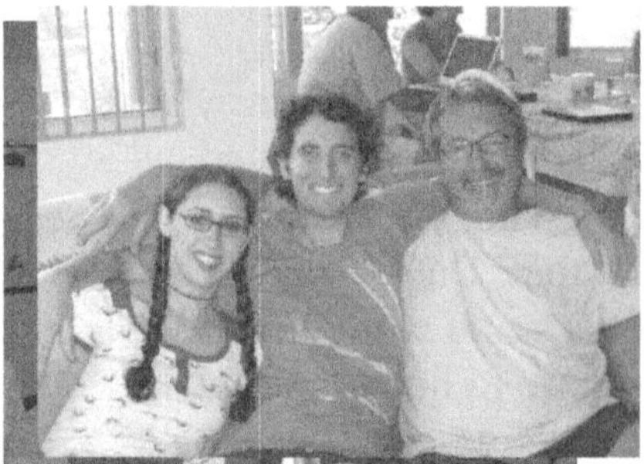

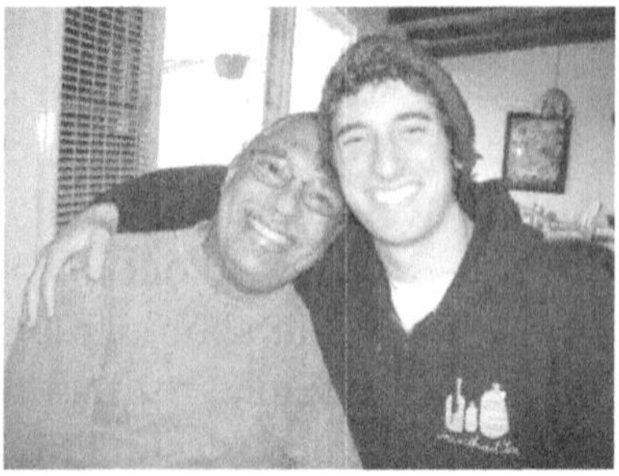

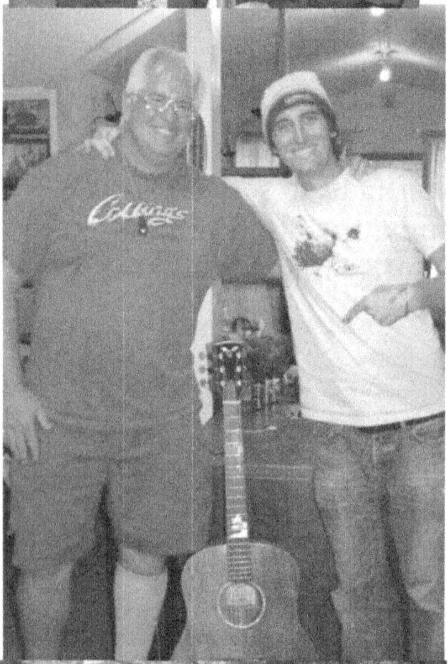
Collings

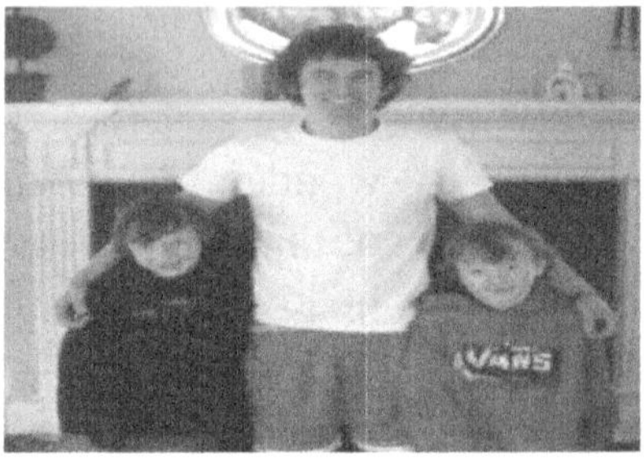
VANS

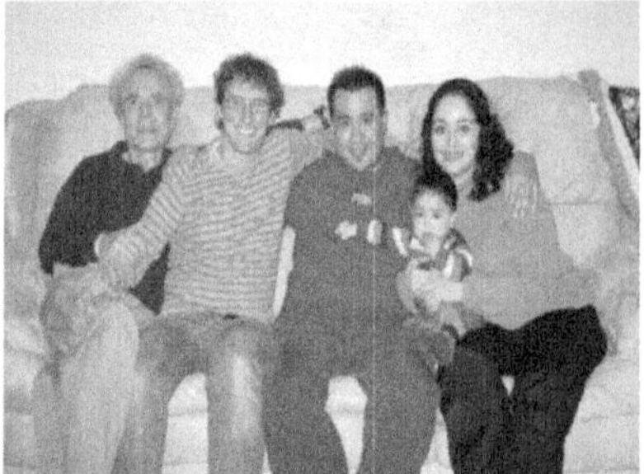

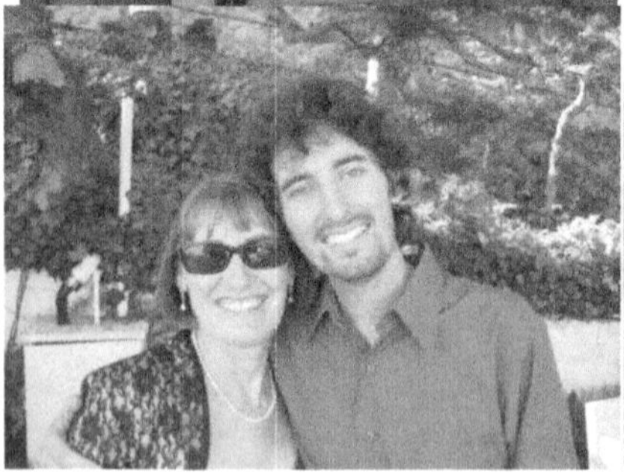

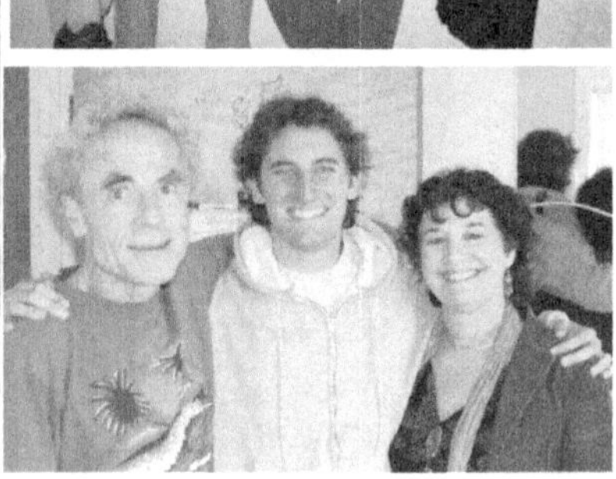

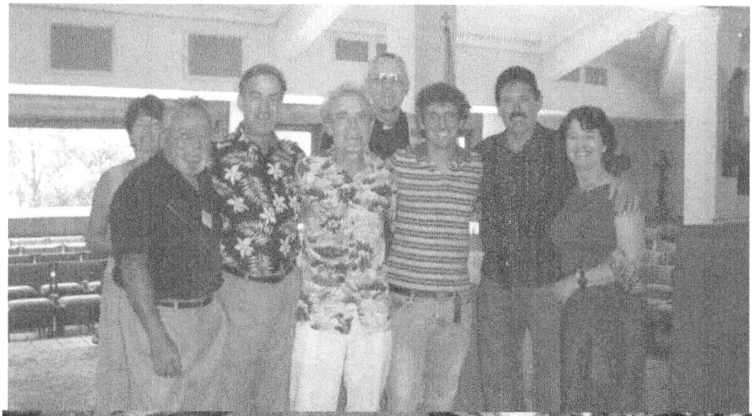

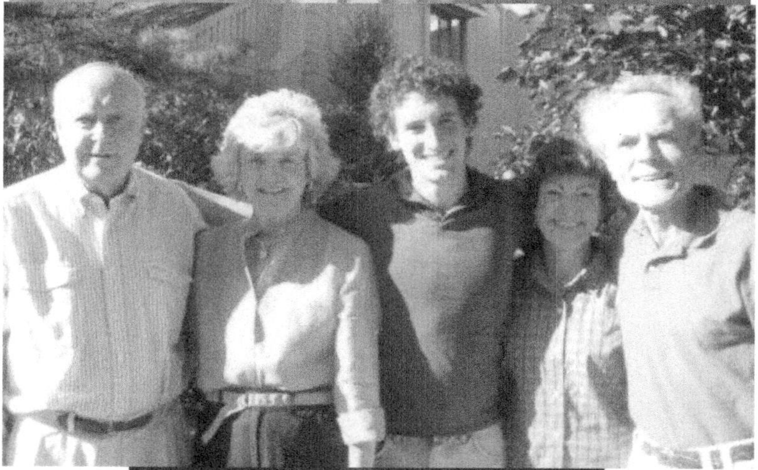

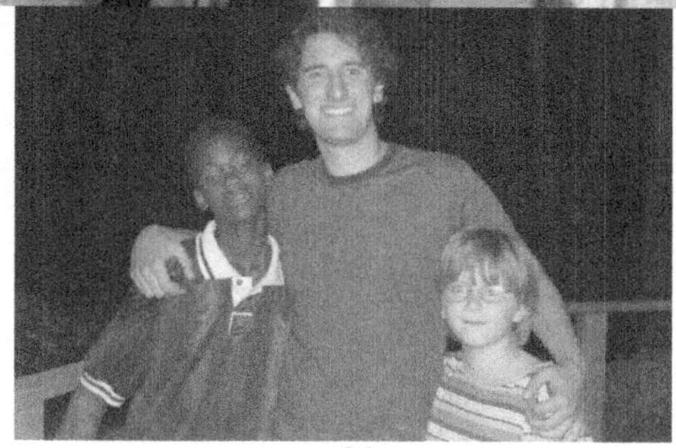

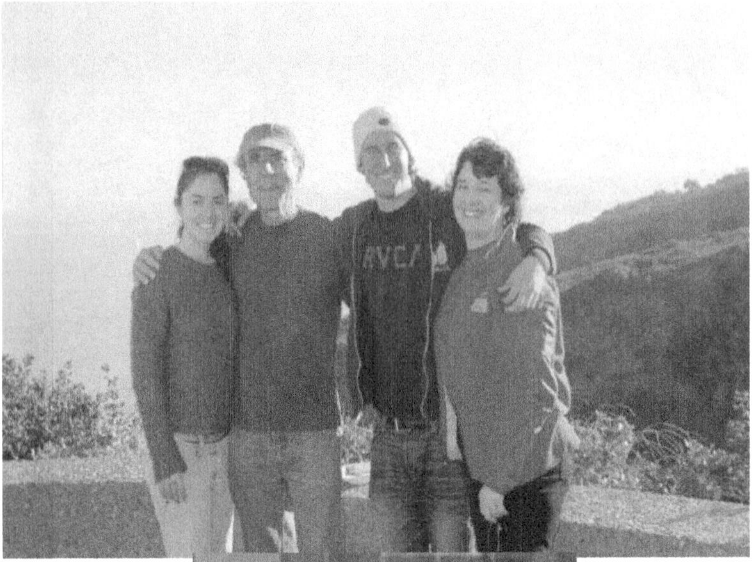

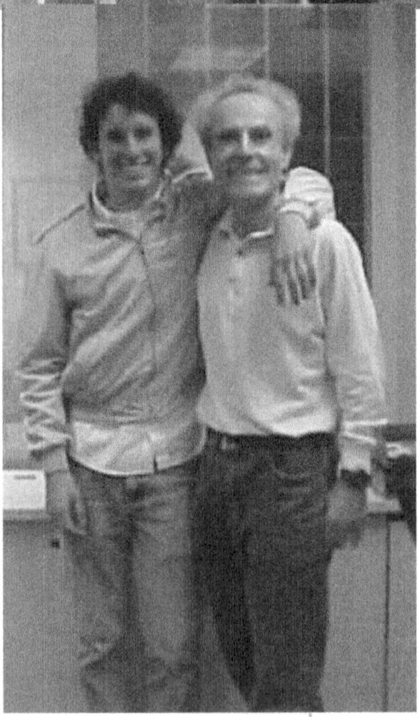

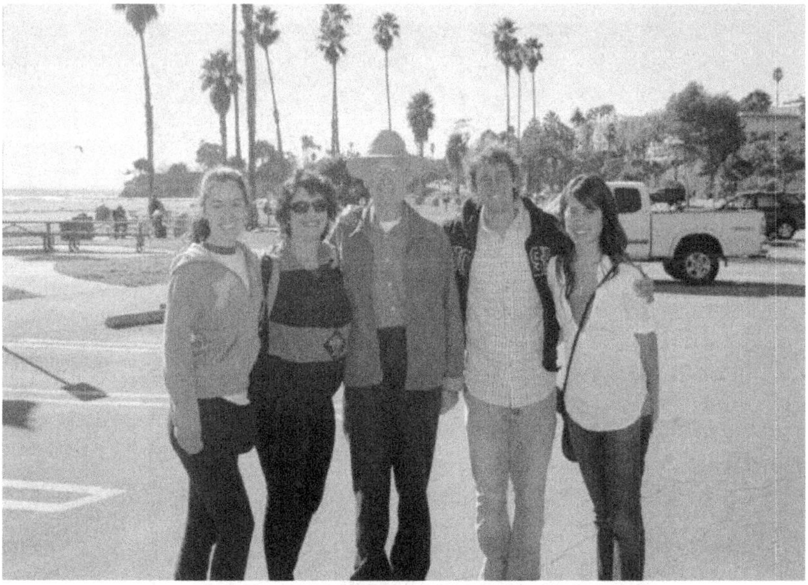

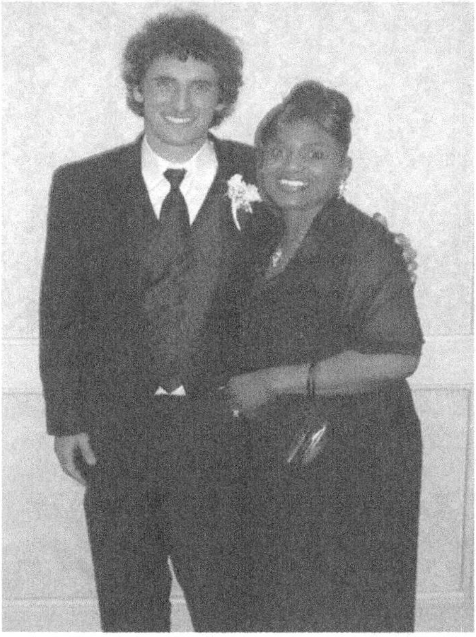

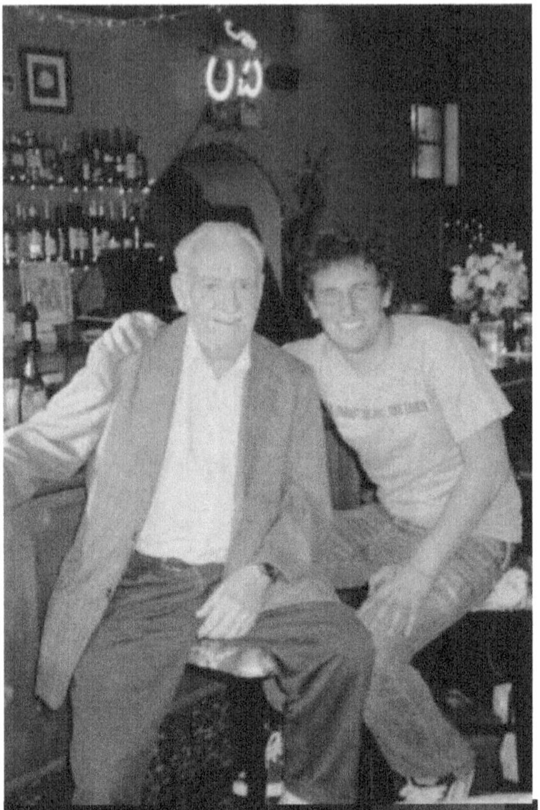

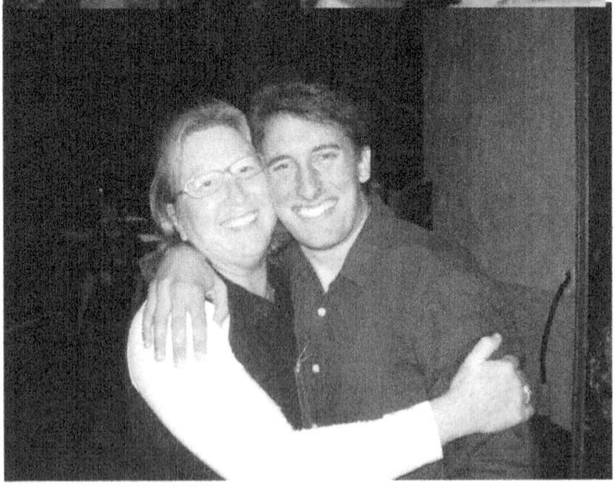

13
Eyes

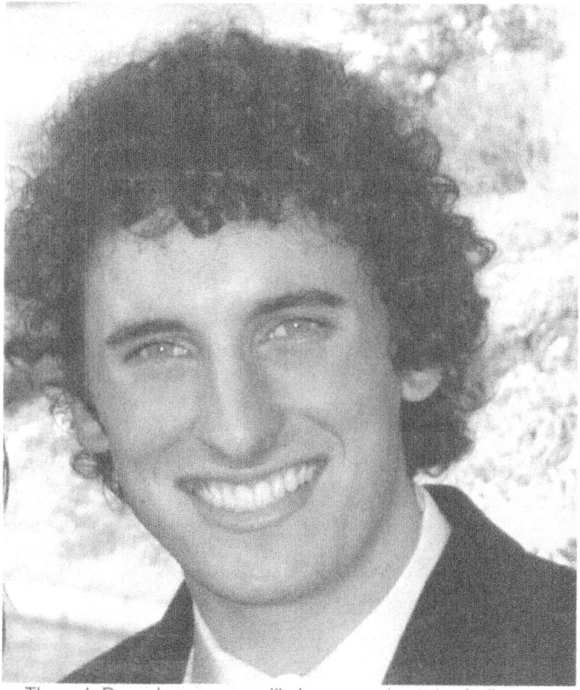

Through Danny's eyes, we will always see hope in challenges. Through his spirit, we feel joy despite pain. And through his music, we continue to share his love and wisdom.

Danny had beautiful blue eyes that guided him throughout his almost twenty years, taking in life's simple and complex realities. He became an avid reader so his eyes also consumed books. He loved the written word and hoped to be more skilled at sharing his love of writing with others, particularly in the lyrics of his songs. What I would call his "signature" song "Through Their Eyes" is about eyes taking in the view of life as others see it:

> I wake up each morning and take a look around.
> My eyes are so tired, I can hardly see.
> And then I notice the reminder above my door:
> Not to forget the ones I adore.
>
> I need to remember to take it from their side,
> and think of things through their minds.
> I need to remember to take it from their side,
> and look at things through their eyes.
>
> So wait a moment, before your throw that fist,
> or scratch another name off your list.
> The whole world doesn't rotate just for you.
> You have to think about the others too.
>
> I need to remember to take it from their side,
> And think of things through their minds.

I need to remember to take it from
their side,
and look at things through their eyes.

So if you had to go walking, down
the street in their shoes,
would you think of them in the same
way?
If you had to see things through their
eyes,
would it all be such a surprise?

Danny not only wrote and sang the lyrics of this song he lived them, especially during his brain tumor journey. He was patient with those who cared for him and open to meeting "angels," those whose extra care resonated with his own gentleness and kindness.

While I would give the world to see his eyes gazing at life again, I am thankful that he saw goodness and filtered out the harshness of life through his eyes. He used his eyes to see things in a positive light, and look for love in himself and others.

In a way Danny lives on through his eyes because after his death, Danny's eyes were donated through the One Legacy Foundation, so that others might see .While at the time there was no guarantee that the transplants of his corneas would be successful, we found out years later that this gift that helped two men, one on the east coast and one on the west coast regain their sight. So Danny's eyes are gifts that keep on giving.

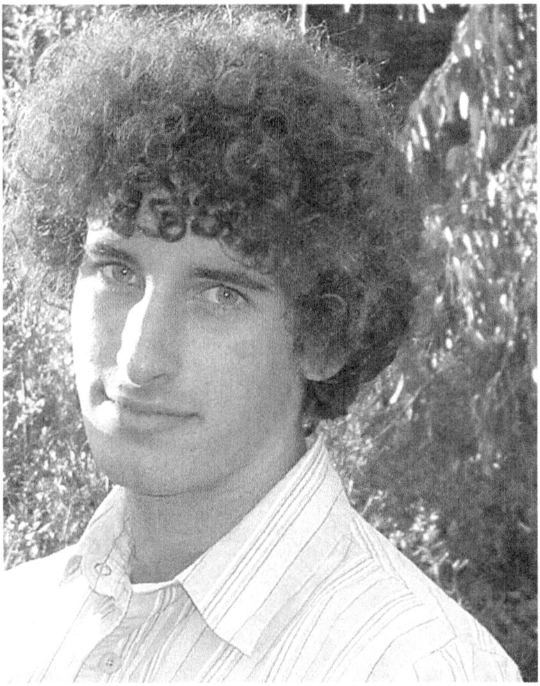

14
Go East Young Man

During spring break of 2006, Danny and I went to Philadelphia for about three weeks to visit family and friends, and to attend my nephew Ed's marriage to Melissa. A few weeks before, Danny had undergone stereotactic radiation surgery for a new lesion on the side of his brain. He was between treatments and feeling pretty good. Certainly his spirits were high, which was not unusual.

We made plans to see the musical "Phantom of the Opera" on Broadway. Beyond wanting to see the show, Danny knew that his girlfriend Catherine and her aunt Jessie were also going to see it in New York about the same time. While it did not work out that we were there together, Danny figured he would surprise Catherine with a letter, which she would hopefully find, planted somewhere in the city otherwise known as the "big apple." I learned about this scheme of his on the plane heading to Philly. I noticed Danny writing a letter and asked who it was for. He proudly replied that it was for Catherine, that he was going to leave it for her in New York City because she and her Aunt Jessie would be there the week after we saw the show. "Leave a letter somewhere in New York City and Catherine would find it?" thought his cynical old man. Danny shared none of my doubt, so he kept writing his letter, which would get a "special delivery."

In the busy-ness of visiting family and making arrangements to stay at my nephew George's house for our New York trip, I forgot about the letter. Unfortunately, Danny did too which I found out as he let out an expletive on the way up in the car. He forgot to bring the letter! As they say, "the best laid plans." Since we were to go right to the show, he had to exercise Plan B once we got there. We had tickets, but still had to wait awhile outside the theater. During that time, Danny went exploring for paper and pen and returned with a cheap pen and oversized post card.

When we were seated, he wrote Catherine a note, a replacement for the long letter, but integral to his plan to leave her something to "find" from him in the big city. Once the wonderful show was over, Danny was a "man on a mission" to place the note somewhere where Catherine could get it when she came to the same show a week later. I thought about Will-Call, but that could only be for the next show. Then, the crazy ideas started to flow from Danny: under a chair, behind a sign outside the theater, at the cashier's in the theater or maybe a store or restaurant nearby… While I felt this was a futile effort, I encouraged my son, the ever positive romantic. Walking down the street, he spotted the entrance to the subway with the grates on three sides of the descending stairs. Bingo, Danny's blue eyes lit up and his warm smile returned! He folded it and put it in the corner of the railing of the entrance, which was at 44nd and 8th Street. Confident that he could give her clues to find it, he placed it there gently, but with firmness of purpose and pleasure. He even took a picture, which I think he sent as a clue.

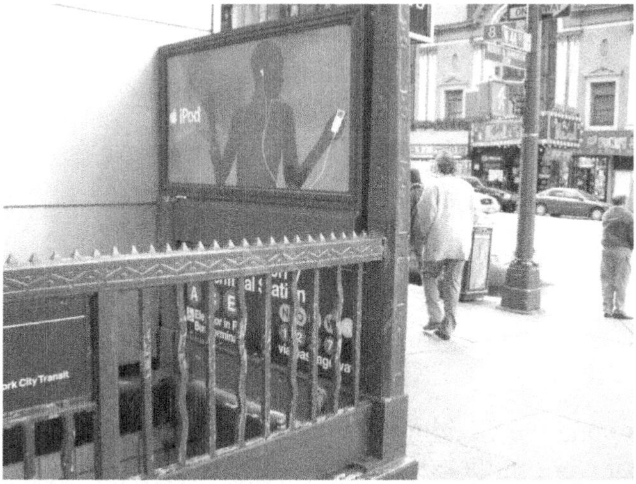

About a week later, when we were at the wedding reception, Danny got a call from Catherine, who was in New York. Yep! With Aunt Jessie's help, she found the note. Danny told me he knew she would!

Speaking of the wedding reception, Danny sang his song "Weeping Willow" at it, dedicating it to Ed and Melissa, the newlyweds. It's one of his love songs, which fit the occasion and he sang it beautifully. The reaction of those present reflected Danny's life at the time. Half the room, the Gibson/ Riley family, was in tears because they knew of Danny's medical condition, the other half seemed to be amazed at his talent and what the future might hold for his sharing it. Danny focused on the present, even singing with the band.

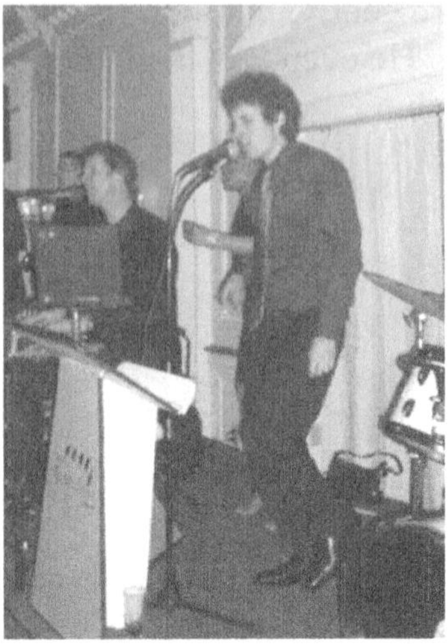

Beyond the wedding there were other family events that were fun. One was the 76 ers (Philly's Pro Basketball Team) game. My nephew Mike Riley arranged to have a luxury box for the family, who came to join Danny at his first Pro game (mine as well). Mike even arranged for Danny to go down on the floor before the game to meet the players. While Danny did not usually like any special attention, he enjoyed it that day and spoke about it thereafter.

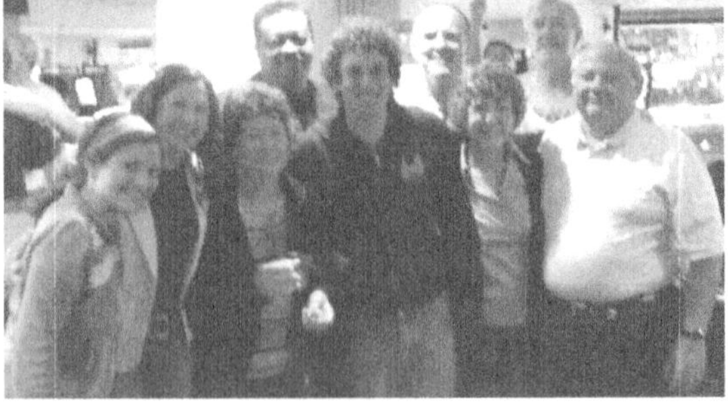

When Maggi, Danny, and I were back East in the Fall of 2005 on a trip that was mainly to Boston for our nephew Joey's marriage to Kaitlyn, we came to Philly and stayed at my brother Tom and his wife Sheila's house. The Wissahickan, a nature trail next

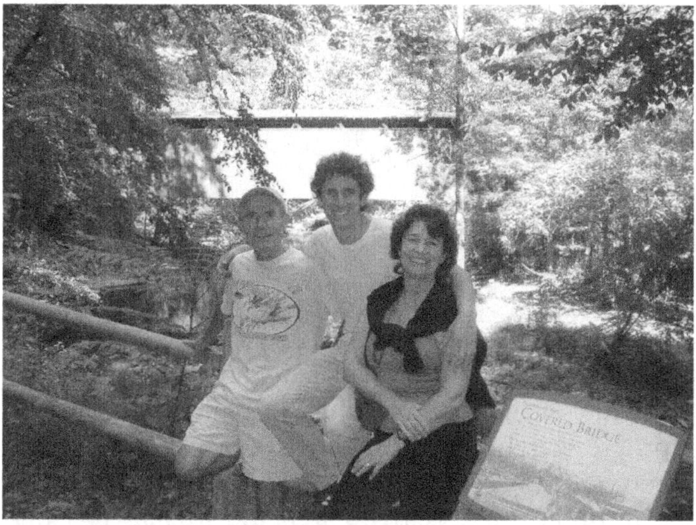

to the river/creek of the same name, where we took Danny for a hike, is a short drive from their house. When we returned this time, Danny wanted to go there again to enjoy it in the Spring. Maggi joined us in Philly later on in our trip, so she was there for our visit to the Wissahickan, taking pictures of Danny exploring its trails. We asked a passerby to take a photo of the three of us by the covered bridge, dating back to the 1800s

15
Words

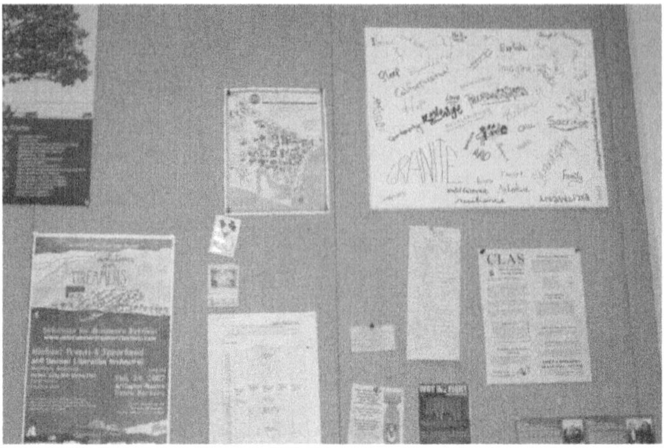

Words were important to Danny and certain words became even more meaningful as his cancer progressed. In the summer of 2006, as he was getting ready to head to the University of California, Santa Barbara, to begin college, he came up with the idea to ask selected family and friends to put just one word on a white canvas board. I don't know who put the first word, but I was among that group and added the word "Hope." The words that Danny's friends and family put on the board ranged from inspirational to funny, but all felt close to Danny because he asked them to join in his project.

One of the last persons to write on the board was Fr. Dave Austin, a family friend who was visiting from Australia late August 2007 and stayed in Danny's room because Danny was in the hospital at the time.

Dave noticed the board in Danny's room, and I went ahead and asked him to write a word on it. Later, when I looked at the board, I saw three new words: "moments of grace." When Danny got out of the hospital and learned that I had asked Dave to write on the board, he was upset with me because it was his board and he was the only one to ask people. And then he found out that Dave had written three words! As was usual with Danny, he later said: "Poppy, it's okay, I would have asked Dave and the words are nice." I referred to these words at the memorial service, that many of our times together especially toward the end of Danny's journey were "moments of grace," precious times filled with the pain and joy life sometimes gives us at the same time, etching memories in our hearts.

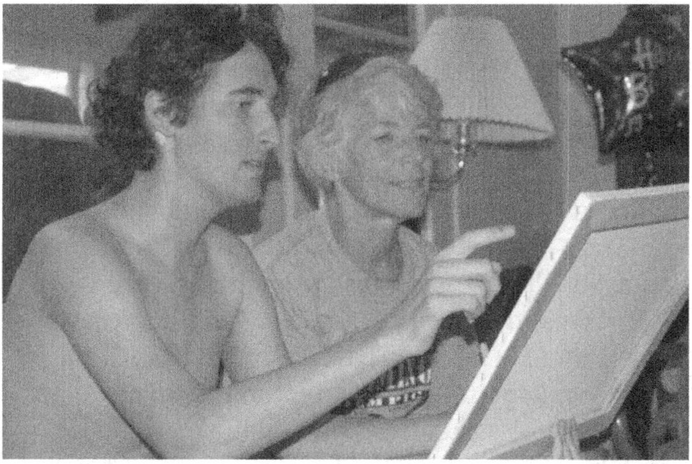

Danny invites Mrs. Hirakawa (his favorite elementary teacher) to sign the board.

16
Circles

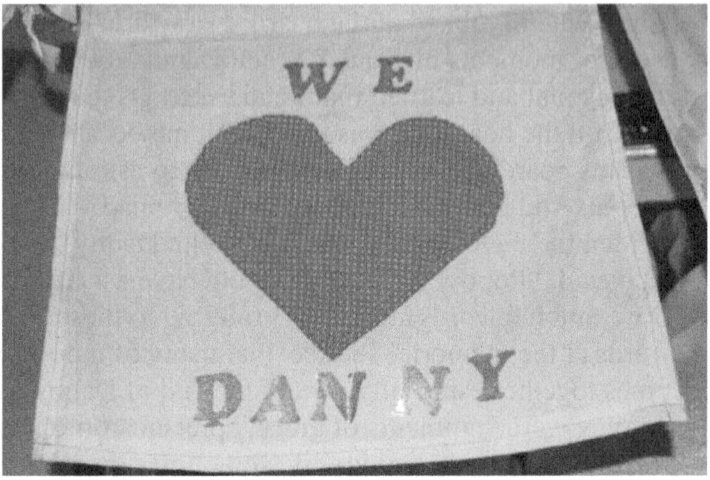

Danny's story can only be understood by an appreciation of the circles of love and life that surrounded him: circles that extended beyond his family and close friends to others who happened to know someone who loved him or learned about his battle with brain cancer. The circle of love that touched Danny deeply during his journey included his large extended family on both coasts: grandpa, aunts, uncles, cousins, his godmother, Tonie Brucelas and her family and his godfather, Joe Dibos and his family. There were circles within circles, inner circles, and an intimate one made up of those who surrounded him on the morning he took his last breath. All who made up these various and intertwined circles graced Danny's life and he always wanted to let them know that:

when i speak these words my tounge gets tied and my knees buckle. youre oh so kind! where can a tribute begin to commend you for all the troubles and thoughts youve spent on such a distant cause and for my sake, ill always remember and always take, you with me in my heart.

--Danny

Central to Danny's inner circle of love were his mother, sister, myself, and Catherine, the young woman he come to know and love in his junior year of high school. Catherine Omalev-Estrada was the love of his life and made Danny's life a true "Love Story." She was in the intimate circle during his last days and final moments of life sharing her love and elegant presence. As Danny would go in and out of consciousness, he was always asking in his words and eyes: "Where's Catherine?" and there she was! She is an amazing young woman from a wonderful family, which Danny became a part of in the final years of his life. Her family joined us in San Francisco for his last operation, and supported him and us in the final days, hours of his life, and are part of our extended family.

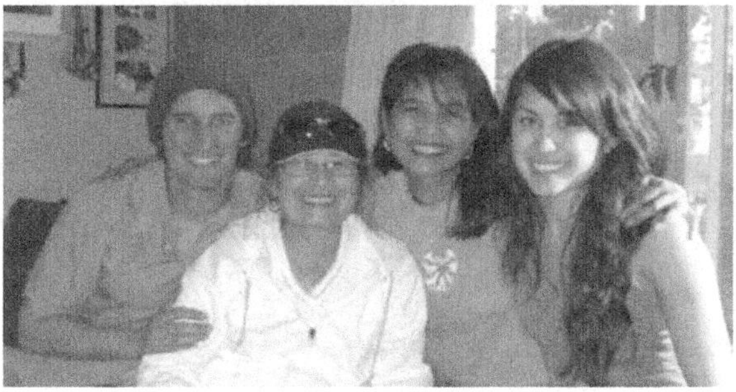

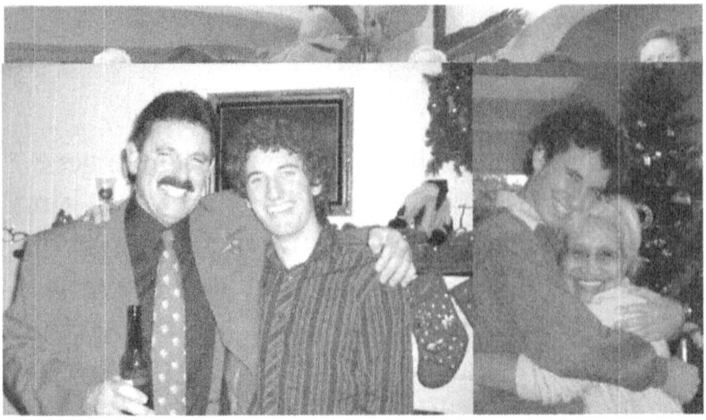

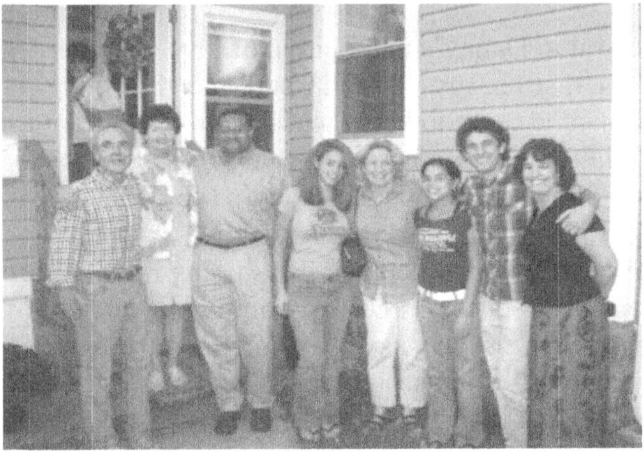

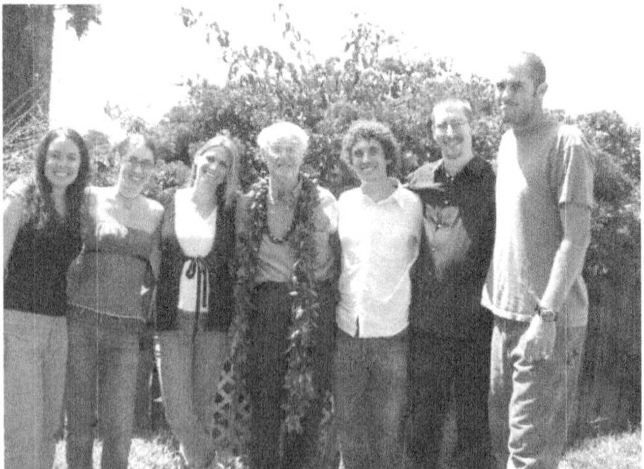

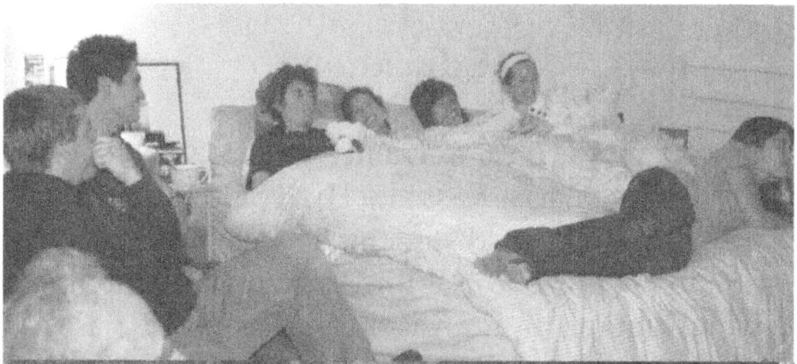

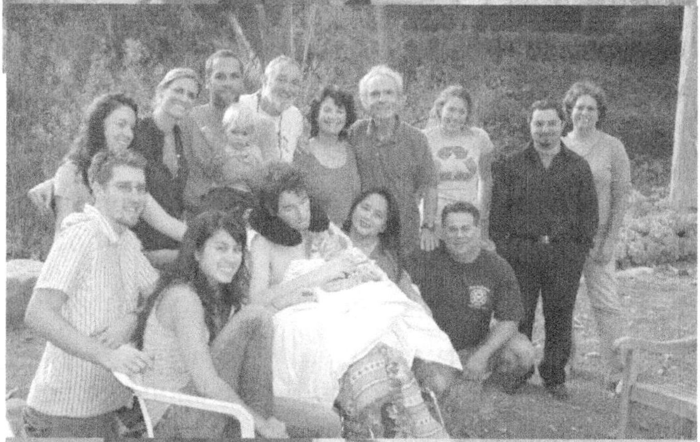

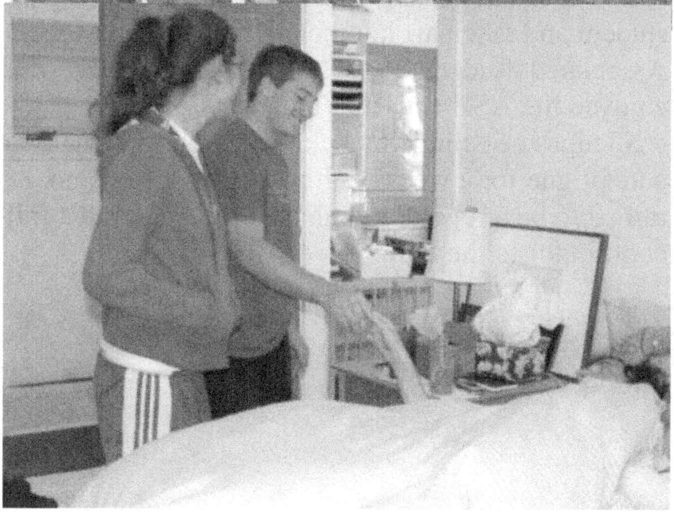

17
Education

Learning was central to Danny's story, which began in his junior year at Eastlake High School in Chula Vista. Always a good student, he was hitting his stride in his third year at this large public school. He took advantage of the Advanced Placement classes (AP) that were available and had his eyes set on attending a good college, maybe even Stanford, where his sister was going. He took part in sports at school, cross-county, track, and soccer. On December 7, 2004, he played left defender in the Varsity soccer game that Eastlake lost to Bonita Vista, their arch rival. I was there as I was for most of his games.

While the discovery of the brain tumor on December 8, 2004 ended his participation in school sports, it did not change his desire to be an excellent student and take part in other activities such as the Associated Student Body (ASB). Danny really enjoyed the ASB activities and despite the challenges of being almost knocked out with nausea and fatigue for a week each month by the chemo, he rallied to be a regular member of his class and a full contributor to the ASB.

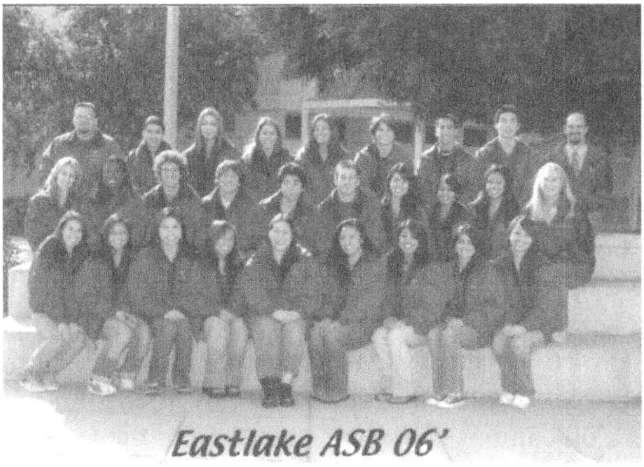

As he wrote in the college application essay,
he had to drop some classes due to the treatments,
but he was able to graduate with his Class in 2006,
with excellent grades and high AP scores
to bring to college.

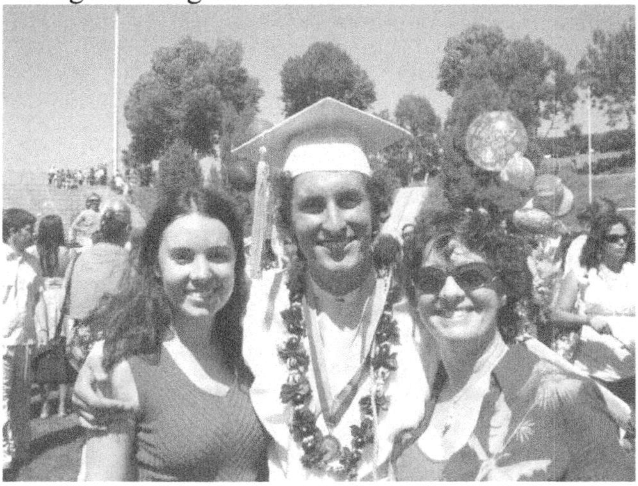

The proud graduate with his mother and sister.

Danny chose to become a University of California Santa Barbara (UCSB) "Gaucho" for many reasons, but mostly because his cousins had graduated from the school, Catherine was going there, and he loved Santa Barbara. We were concerned about the lack of a big hospital in the area, but were able to arrange for him to receive his various treatments at the Cancer Center of Santa Barbara. Dr. Elizabeth Downing at the UCSB Student Health Center generously reached out to support, monitoring him with weekly visits and special arrangements for lab work on campus. With assistance from the UCSB Center for Students with Disabilities, Danny was able to complete his freshman year with honors, despite a second brain surgery in March.

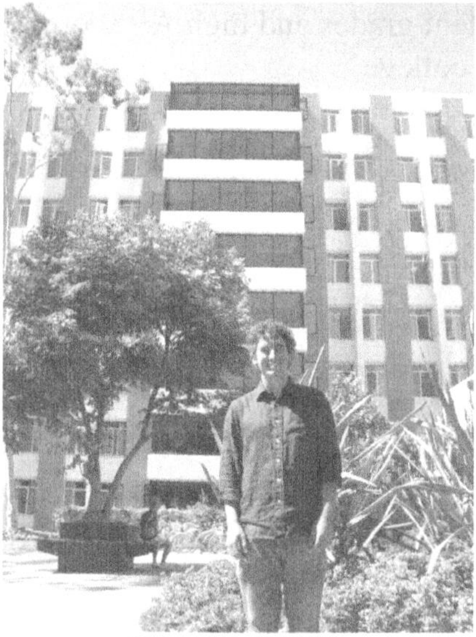

Danny at UCSB

The summer of 2007 was a rough one for him, in and out of the hospital and the Cancer Center of San Diego for nausea, hydration and pain management due to brain tumor growth. His condition became so bad that the only option was a third and final brain surgery, which we were able to have done at UCSF Medical Center. So, in mid-August he had to be flown by air ambulance to San Francisco for his third craniotomy.

Even though he was drained due to the ongoing nausea and pain (and his prognosis was dire because there was no further treatment), Danny was determined to return to UCSB and enrolled in a full load of classes for the Fall semester of his sophomore year and even lived for a short time in an apartment in Isla Vista with five of his buddies.

With the help of Visiting Nurses and Hospice of Santa Barbara, who provided almost daily in-home support, he went to class until October 11, 2007, by bike, no less. However, on that day he had to be helped back to his apartment by Dr. Downing, the vigilant campus doctor whose care enabled him to go to school as long as he could. That evening, he was driven to his Uncle Darryl's birthday party at Kim and Jack Johnson's house in Santa Barbara, where he remained until he died 20 days later. He pursued his education as long as possible.

Danny was a member of the Class of 2010, so I wrote this at the time of the graduation of his college classmates:

Class of 2010

At this time of year, seniors at various university campuses participate in that wonderful rite of passage called college graduation. Students, buoyed by the support of their families, set their sights on this event four years ago with the hopes and promises it held. For most parents, this is a time of pride even as they face the financial investment they made to support their son or daughter's achievement. The fear of "letting-go," when they dropped off their teenagers at the campus four years ago is replaced by the sense of pride they see in their now mature and independent graduates.

My feelings about the Class of 2010 are colored by the absence of my son Danny who should be among those graduating. When Danny started college at the University of California at Santa Barbara in September of 2006, the month of June 2010 represented a hope for not only graduation, but for life, as he had been diagnosed with brain cancer in 2004. While Danny will not line up among the young men and women receiving diplomas from UCSB this year, he will always be a member of the Class of

2010 because he gave his all to be a vibrant part of it, even biking to class just twenty days before he died on October 31, 2007. Despite on-going chemotherapy and another brain surgery during his freshman year, Danny completed the year on the Dean's List.

In September of 2007, Danny started his sophomore year, even though he had a third surgery in August and a dire prognosis. He returned to UCSB to be with his friends and experience all that goes with college life. He wanted to live off-campus in the apartment he and his friends had lined-up before summer break. Danny chose to live in the midst of the challenges that a college environment brings. Most of all, like other young people, he wanted to prepare for the future by living the demands of the present: classes, assignments, deadlines, all-nighters, parties, etc. Danny's future was his present. In his application essay for the UC system, he wrote: "Whatever time I may lose out on in the future, I am sure to make up for by living now." For Danny, that meant being an active member of the Class of 2010, as long as he could.

As prominent commencement speakers inspire the members of the Class of 2010 to live their dreams and be leaders of tomorrow, perhaps the most challenging words are those of their classmate:

> Live a life that is hard working and
> true to yourself.
> Seek that which you desire;
> Offer that which life inspires.
> Recognize the beauty of life and
> repay this gift, through
> the care you take in living well.
> Then, life will repay you
> for the services you've granted it.
>
> -Danny

Danny's academic achievements were recognized, especially in high school. He received many awards and scholarships which he was really proud of and helped him in his applications for college. Below is a picture of him receiving one accompanied by Christina Robles, his counselor, who was a big reason he was able to do so well in high school and be accepted at all the colleges he applied to, eventually choosing the University of California, Santa Barbara.

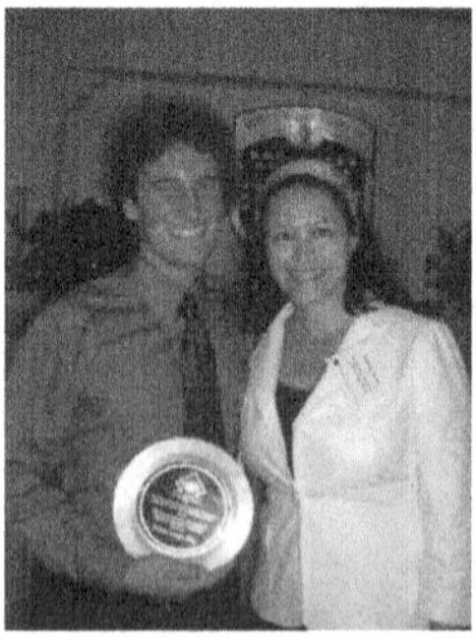

18
300,000 Miles

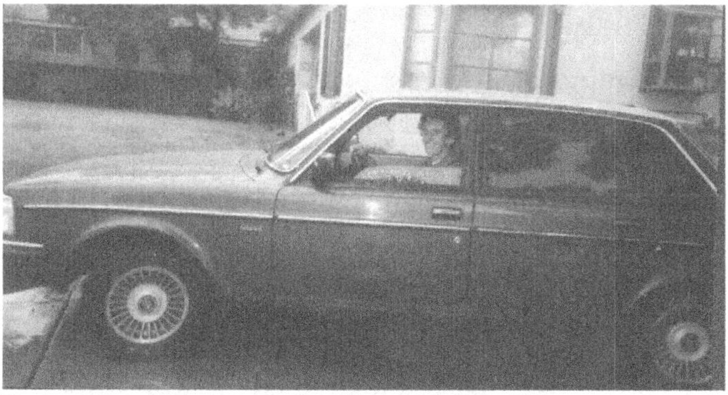

Danny turned sixteen in December of his sophomore year of high school, so he was one of the first of his class to drive. It was a trying time for his parents, but thrilling for him. He took the responsibility seriously and took care of the car we provided for him, an old Volvo that used to be his sister's. From the time he got the car, he had the goal of driving it to the 300,000 mile mark, which he fell short of by about three thousand miles. The year after he died we drove it over that threshold in his honor. Danny did drive it for many miles and good uses: high school, one year of college at UC Santa Barbara, treatments throughout those three years, concerts, get-togethers, and to the places he loved, especially Catherine's house.

He usually picked up friends on his way to high school, except when he was too sick and I was his substitute. One of his passengers was Emmercelle, who wrote about the trips in an essay for her college

newspaper (University of California, Irvine
February 17, 2009 **My Best Friend Died of Cancer**
By Emmercelle Deleon):

Daniel Joseph Riley and his maroon Volvo waited for me every morning at 6:30 a.m. Although I would always ask for five more minutes when he'd call, twenty-five minutes later we'd be on our way to Eastlake High School. He never once complained. Opening his car door, music would hit me – Elliott Smith, Damien Rice, or, if I was lucky, KC and Jojo. "Allllll myyy liiiiiiife," Daniel wouldwail, "I prayed for someone liiiiike youuuuu," his thumbs drummingon the plastic steering wheel, his brown curly hair bobbing to keep time with the music…Between concerts, student government and shared classes, inside Daniel's car we had our personal psychiatric sessions. Mentally and emotionally everyday Daniel took me home. Clad in glasses and his favorite "Me Without You" jacket, Daniel was the-know-it-all and the "I do speak for everyone when I say ... " on a variety of topics, from boyfriends with outrageous laughs to why I didn't win the school election when my other two running mates did. " You did the best you could do, and that should be enough for you," Daniel told me, and didn't say anything when I accidentally let a tear slip.-

Danny loved the '86 Volvo, which seemed to be "reciprocal" because it got him to his doctor's appointments, radiation and chemo treatments, even to the hospital in Santa Barbara when he was in severe pain.

My late brother Ed and I accompanied Danny on a trip from Santa Barbara. In December 2006, we went up by train and returned with him on his drive back to Chula Vista because I did not want him to drive that distance alone. The trip was a lot of fun, full of jokes, and stories, mostly involving Ed, one of Danny's favorite uncles. On Danny's urging, I retold the "There's Eddie!" story, which was even more fun because the main character in it was present in the car. Briefly, it's about Eddie's surprise presence in New York City one New Year's Eve. Ed was just turning 18 and asked my dad to borrow the car, a 1947 Hudson, to go to a local party near our home in a suburb of Philadelphia, about 90 miles from New York City. As was our custom, those who were home watched Dick Clark at Times Square to bring in the new year, which I think was 1953. As a ten year old, I was fascinated with the dropping of the ball, so I zeroed in on the crowd waiting for it to drop. As I was watching, I thought I saw Eddie's curly hair and big smile and yelled out: "There's Eddie." By the time I got the attention of my parents and siblings, Dick and Jean, the scene had changed and Eddie was not there. But when the ball started descending and we all focused on the crowd at the foot of it, sure enough: There was Eddie! So, sometimes Ed's presence would bring crazy surprises, but in the car on that trip home from Santa Barbara it brought plenty of Danny's roaring laughs.

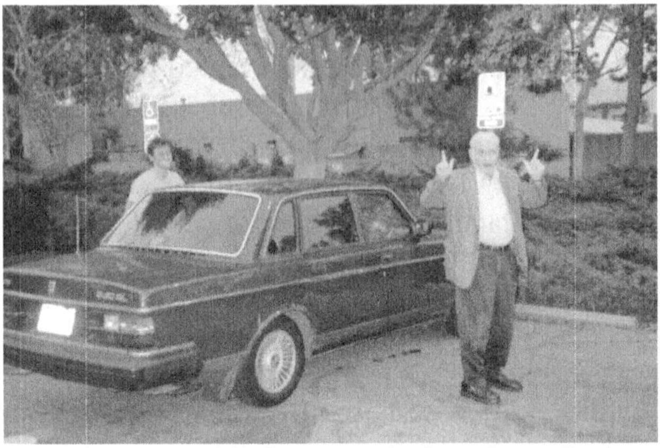

Ed goofing around before our trip from Santa Barbara.

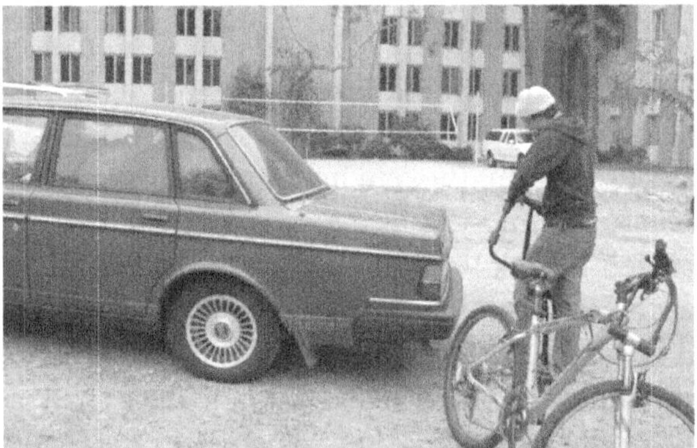

Danny was on his bike or in his car until October 11, 2007.

Danny only had one accident during his short driving career. It consisted of backing out of a friend's driveway into a car, parked on a narrow street. This may be symbolic because Danny was always looking forward: to a new day, a new song, learning something new, making new friends, closer relationships with others, and driving his beloved maroon Volvo over the 300,000 mile mark.

19
“Make That 56!”

When Danny had his second brain surgery in March of 2007 at the UC Medical Center in San Francisco, the surgeon made the incision from his hairline in front all the way to the nape of his neck in the back and closed it up with metal staples. About a week later, before we traveled back to U.C. Santa Barbara, another neurosurgeon removed the 55 staples with gentle care. Danny was fascinated by the large number of staples and joked about the process of removing them. He even posed for pictures so his friends and family could see them.

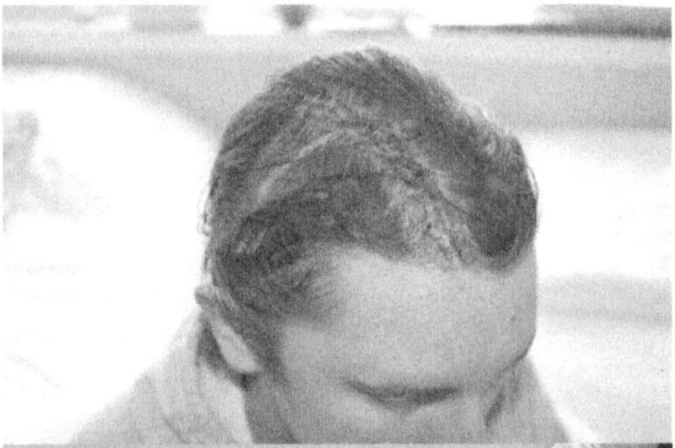

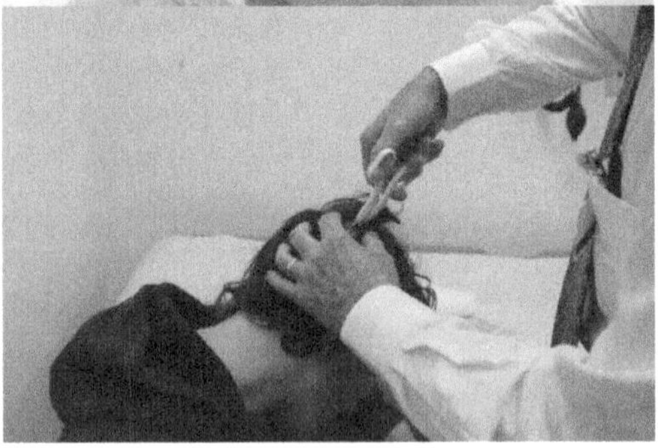

Danny's jovial mood about the staples was evident on the trip to Santa Barbara. I was driving when Maggi received a call from her brother Ron. Talking about the operation, she mentioned that he had 55 staples put in his scalp to close the incision. While rubbing the back of his head, Danny overheard this and shouted out "Make that 56!" The doctor had missed one. Later he had it removed in Santa Barbara. Danny returned to his dorm, resumed his studies, and began a new regimen of chemo at the Cancer Center of Santa Barbara. In August, he had to have another craniotomy which required a similar incision and staples. This time the surgery was not filled with the same optimism about the future as the previous one was, but Danny's demeanor did not reflect that. He joked with the doctor about missing one staple the time before.

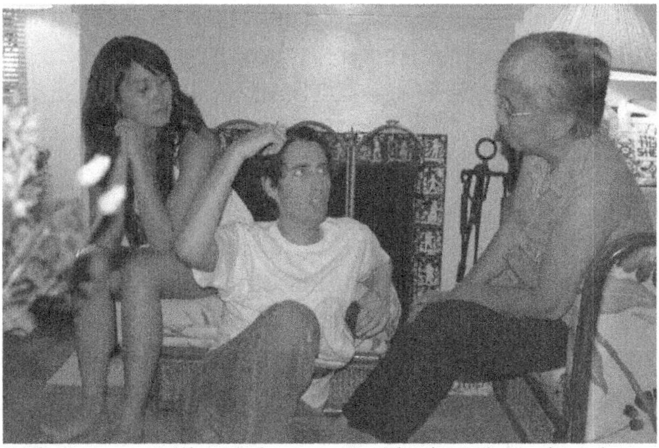

When we got back home to Chula Vista, he showed his godmother Tonie the scar and told her that this time they got all the staples

20
No Harm, No Foul

Anyone who has ever played a game of "pick-up" basketball, where there are no refs, knows the expression: "No harm, no foul," which means that even if you get hit, tripped, or otherwise fouled but keep going, no foul is called. This expression applies to Danny's story because there were some problems along the way. One was discovered by Maggi in reviewing his chemo treatments in Santa Barbara. The otherwise excellent physician miscalculated the dosages for the two chemo agents and had them reversed. Maggi discovered this after several months of treatment had occurred. When Danny found out about it, his concern was if there was any proof of negative consequences, known bad effects. At the time, it was uncertain. So, his response was: "No harm, no foul," and he just kept on going with the revised treatment plan and hope for positive effects. He never blamed the doctor, nor thought any less of him.

During Danny's second brain surgery, he had to have a synthetic piece of material put in to replace the cancer-ridden section of his dura matter, the thin covering of the brain, that had to be removed. While the operation was a success in terms of what they could do for Danny, a few weeks later he received a letter indicating that there was a recall of the synthetic material that had been put into his head. When you hear recall, you usually think of a part of a car or appliance, that can be easily replaced, not something already inside your head. Fortunately, Danny's neurosurgeon, Dr. Nolin Gupta at UCSF Medical Center, was very reassuring telling us that the chances of infection were slight and how to monitor it. Again, Danny's response was: "No harm, no foul."

If there were directives that Danny gave us for his care and treatment, it was to be respectful of all the medical providers and appreciative of their efforts on his behalf. Danny showed us the way. He was always thanking and interacting with nurses, attendants, medical technicians, doctors, social workers, etc. even joking with them.

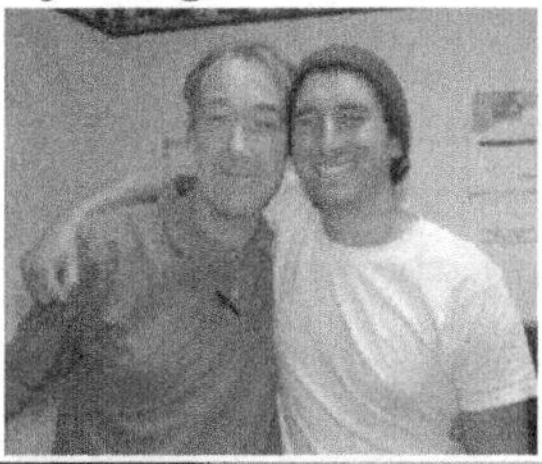

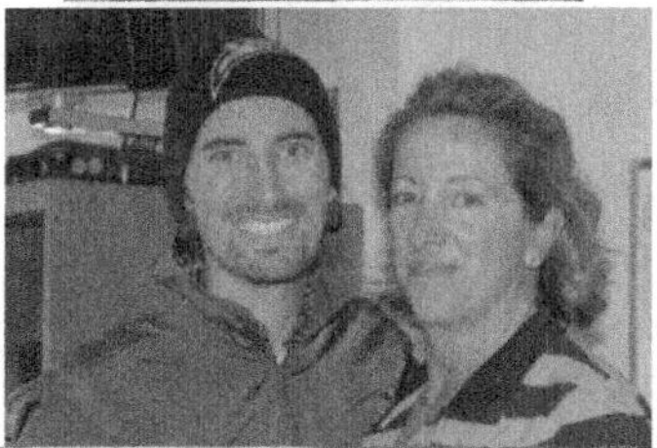

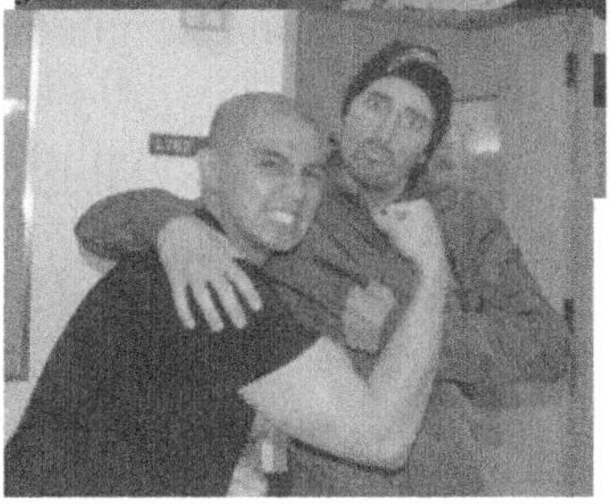

However, there was one exception in the summer of 2007 when he was getting really weak. One doctor, in front of Danny, Maggi, Alicia, and me would not give permission for a test that another doctor had ordered, saying that his condition did not warrant it. This was the only time we really saw Danny upset with a health care provider, especially a doctor. He asked us to see that she was removed from his case, which we immediately arranged. While Danny did not use the expression, this time there was some harm, a real foul was called by him and the referees: Maggi, Alicia, and myself.

If there were another real "foul" that should have been called in Danny's care/story, it would be a "technical foul" against the US Congress for underfunding research to prevent and cure cancer. We learned about the limited number of federally-funded clinical trials, and experienced the difficulty of getting into one at the National Institute of Health in D.C. Our conversations with doctors brought up the theme of a country that spends more on killing than on healing. While we justifiably provide for our national defense against foreign enemies, we spend too little preventing and curing diseases like cancer that are killing our children, sisters, brothers, parents, and neighbors. So, if Danny's story has a lesson it would that we need to speak out "call a foul" when it applies, especially for our government's underfunding of cancer research.

21
The Strength of Others

While there were many influences in Danny's life, one was a good friend of mine, Bill Atkinson. Father Bill Atkinson was a Catholic priest who belonged to the Augustinian Order, known on the East coast for Villanova University. Bill was my friend Al Atkinson's brother. I knew Al from high school and spent summers at Ocean City where Al, Bill, and I played touch football on the beach. Speaking of football, Al went on to play middle linebacker on the Jets team that won the 1969 Super Bowl in a big upset over the Baltimore Colts. A few years earlier Bill joined the Augustinians where I was studying a couple years ahead of him. During his first year in the seminary, Bill has a tragic accident going downhill on a toboggan that left him paralyzed from the neck done. Despite it, Bill went on to become the first quadriplegic priest in the Roman Catholic Church.

While my friendship with Bill predated the Augustinians, it grew stronger during the years we were together and lasted throughout Bill's life which ended September 2006, about a year before Danny's death. Danny met Bill many times during our family trips back East and admired him. When Danny and I went back to Philly for my nephew Ed Gibson's wedding in April 2006, we stopped to visit Bill who was not well. During the visit, Bill asked me to leave the room so he could have some private time with Danny, who was himself suffering from brain cancer. It was not until months later that Danny told me what transpired. He said Bill discussed one of his own poems called: "The Strength of Others." Danny kept a copy by his bed and confided in me how much Bill's words helped him. As I reflect on Bill's life, he was the strength for others, as was Danny.

The Strength of Others

"How'd you do it?" People would say
So confining, day after day
Having others around for constant care
Ever wonder if life's unfair?

"How'd you do it?" People would ask
Is it better now than in the past?
To see others do what you did before
Realizing you cannot do them anymore.

"How'd you do it?" People have said
Needing help in-n-out of bed
Doubts at times? Patience wearing thin?
Ever wonder how it will end?

"How'd you do it?" Day after day
The path taken wasn't my way
The choice was Another's, not my own
He sent me help. Couldn't do it alone.

How'd I do it? Let me confide
Always with others right at my side
Family and friends from the start
Gave me love in no small part.

How'd I do it? Day after day
Would not have it any other way
They shared triumphs and setbacks too
Been blest, when I look back in review.

How'd I do it? Let me reply
On those who help me, I totally relied
They taught me to live, not just to cope
With their love, they gave me hope.

How'd I do it? Day after day
Help of others along the way
Valued friends, sisters and brothers
I simply borrowed-the strength of others.
-- Bill Atkinson

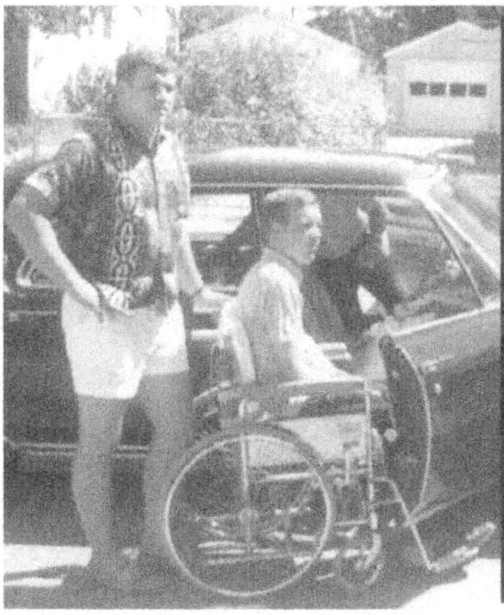
Al and Bill Atkinson, 1969

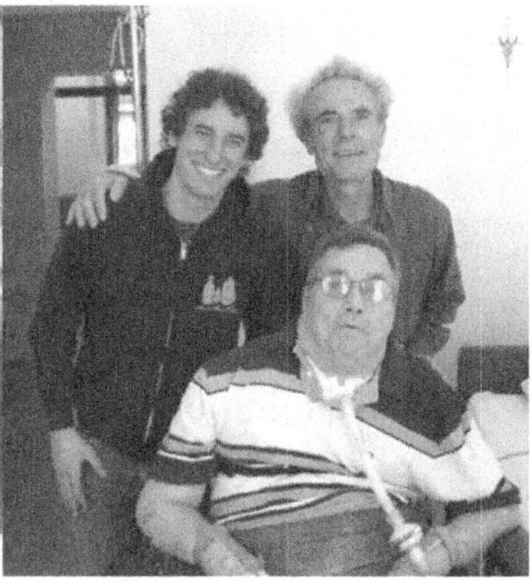
Danny, Frank, and Bill, 2006

22
Big Sur

On the coast of California, between Monterey to the north and San Luis Obispo to the south is an area called Big Sur. It is known for its rugged coast, cypress trees, rolling hills, natural wonders, and breathtaking views of the Pacific Ocean. It has special meaning for our family because the last trip we took together was to Big Sur in June of 2007. After Alicia's graduation from Stanford, we traveled south in two cars but with one mission to spend quality time together as a family in a beautiful part of our state and country.

While we did not know it would be our last trip together, we were aware that it could be and savored every moment. Danny was having more bouts with nausea and pain, but was otherwise able to really enjoy the trip: hike, eat, play his guitar, and be social with us and others.

We stayed at two different lodges, one was famous for its food and guest accommodation, the other was in a State park. Both had access to trails, great views, and gave us time to share as a family. Maggi captured some of the times in beautiful photos, which tell more than I could in words:

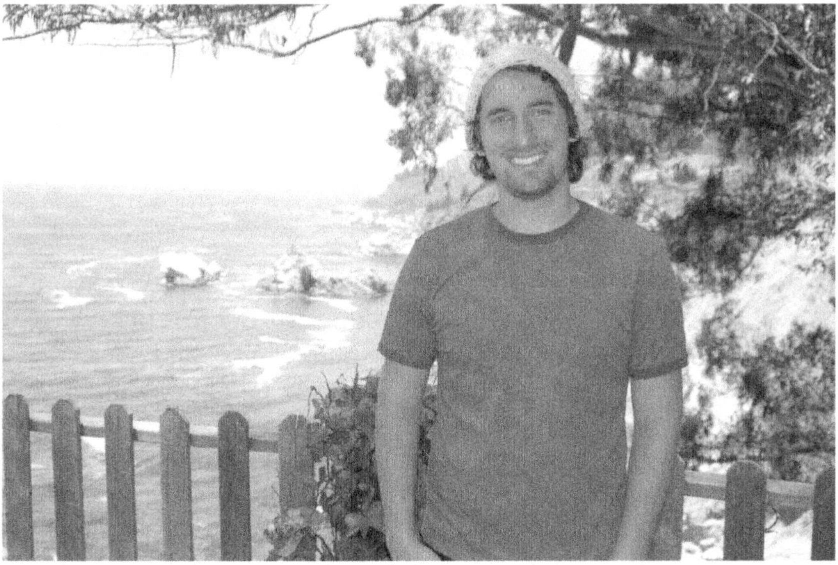

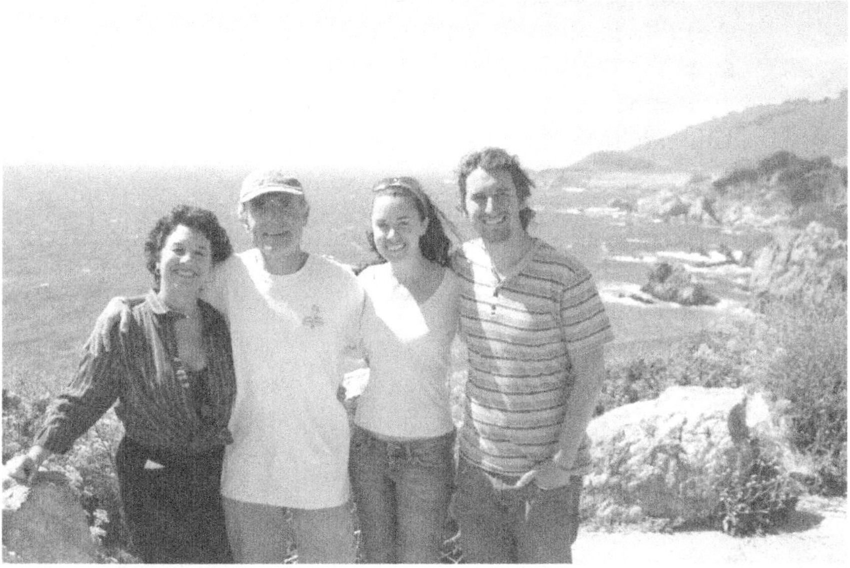

The smiles of Danny with the beauties of nature in the background touched me then and still do as I see him in pictures. Because our family was happy in those June days, Big Sur will always have a special meaning for us. Beyond that, it has taken on a personal one.

Since Danny's death, I decided to go up every year to the New Camaldoli Hermitage in Big Sur to spend a few days in solitude and silence, and plan to keep going as long as I can. Gazing out on the Pacific Ocean, where Danny's ashes have been spread, I appreciate the stillness and rolling waves crashing against the rocks that symbolize life's emotions: the peaceful moments and those that stir the sadness and pain the waves of life can bring. Amid the sounds of nature, I feel the silence of my son. Yet the songs he sang, poetry he wrote, and smiles he shared are still present in the peace that fills the hills, the tides, and whispers of nature.

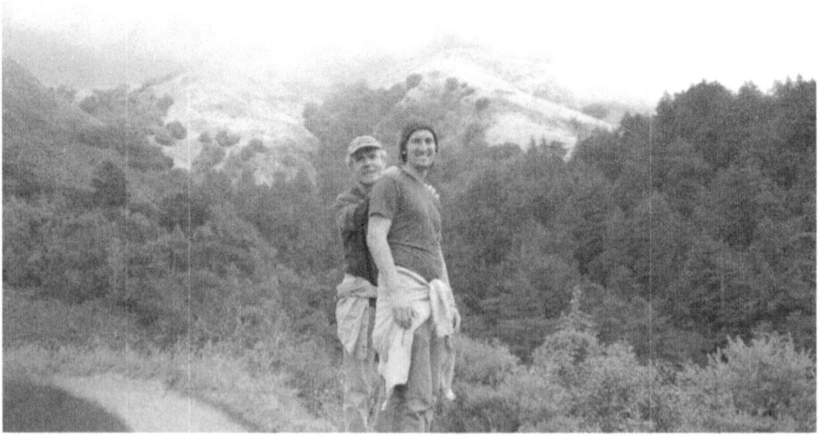

23
The Bachelor Party

Danny loved his cousin Jacob, and the feeling was mutual. As Jacob and Marlo's September 15, 2007 wedding in Santa Barbara approached, Danny grew weaker with constant nausea. Yet, Danny was determined to attend the ceremony on the beach in Santa Barbara and sing at the reception. He wanted to write a special song for them but that eluded him.

Danny and I went up to Santa Barbara early so we could participate in the bachelor party, which was on Thursday morning, a unique time to celebrate the last days of liberty for the about-to-be husband, Jacob. The morning festivities focused on kayaking off the coast of Santa Barbara for a few hours. The 10:00 am start time was tough for Danny but he made it so he could join Jack in the two man kayak (something I had prearranged with Jack). As sick as Danny was leading up to it, he had the time of his (waning) life. He was out on the ocean for about three hours; dolphins swam next to their kayak. It was thrilling for all of us who shared Jacob's last days of bachelorhood. However, it took a toll on Danny. He was at the Cancer Center of Santa Barbara the next day for hydration and was very weak for the Saturday afternoon ceremony and reception. That said, he still managed to gather the strength to sing: "Through Their Eyes," smile, and hug the newly-weds before exiting early.

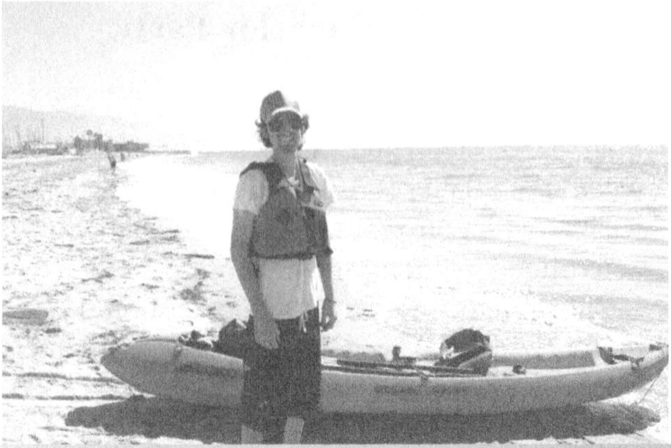

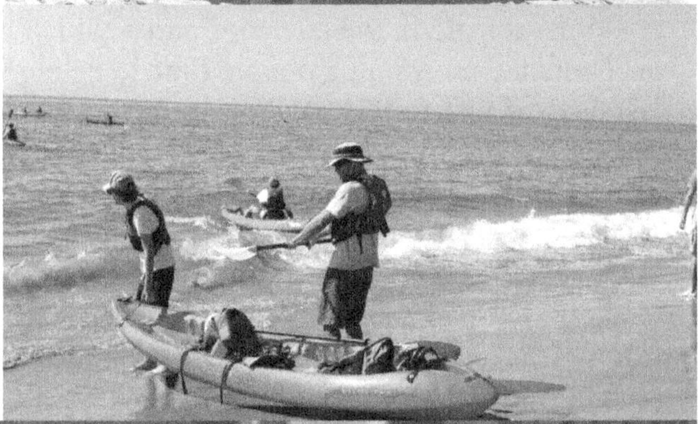

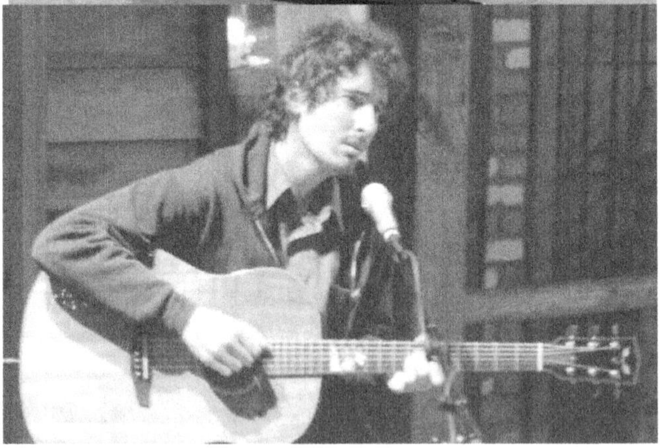

24
Horizon

In mid-August 2007, I knew the horizon of Danny's life was drawing closer, even though I still had hope for a miracle. Yet, even the brightest day has a sunset. Danny's sunset came on October 31, 2007 about eight hours after his last gesture to point to the **LIVESTRONG** bracelet on his wrist. The almost three weeks that he lived at Jack and Kim's house were filled with music, hugs, vigils, camaraderie with him when he could and with each other in between. We laughed, cried, shared our lives as we touched Danny's and he ours. In a sense, I never felt more alive as when Danny was "actively dying," to use the hospice term. In the midst of the sadness there was a deep appreciation of each other and our peaceful /loving connection to Danny Boy: son, brother, nephew, cousin, classmate, friend, who was our strength in his weakness.

The late John O'Donohue, an Irish poet, philosopher, and former priest, has helped me with his poignant writing about life and its ending: the "final horizon."

> The dead are not far away: they are very very near us. Each one of us someday will have to face our own appointment with death. I like to think of it as an encounter with your deepest nature and most hidden self. It is a journey toward a new horizon…death can be understood as the

> final horizon. Beyond there, the deepest well of your identity awaits you. In that well, you will behold the beauty and light of your eternal face.
> **Anam Cara: A Book of Celtic Wisdom,** pp 214-215

Danny's "final horizon," came early in the morning, surrounded by the intimate circle of four, and in spirit the circles of love that were part of his life of almost twenty years. As I wrote in "A Father's Reflection," I was at Danny's side when he took his first breath and his last. Every breath in between was a gift to me and to those who knew and loved him. Like all those who have touched our lives deeply and have crossed this horizon, we want to continue to share their gifts. We long to relive the magic moments we had with them and will always wish for more. We want to go "beyond the horizon," especially after experiencing the death of a young loved one. When Danny died, the intimate circle and Catherine's family, who had come up to be with us, joined in a prayer around Danny's bed. No words can express what the final days were like, but a few discrete pictures may:

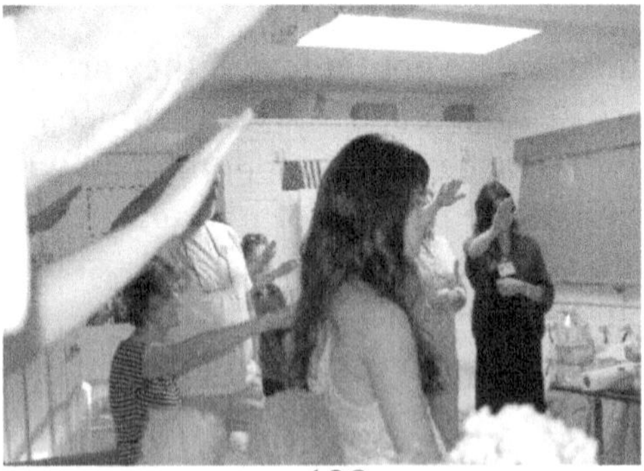

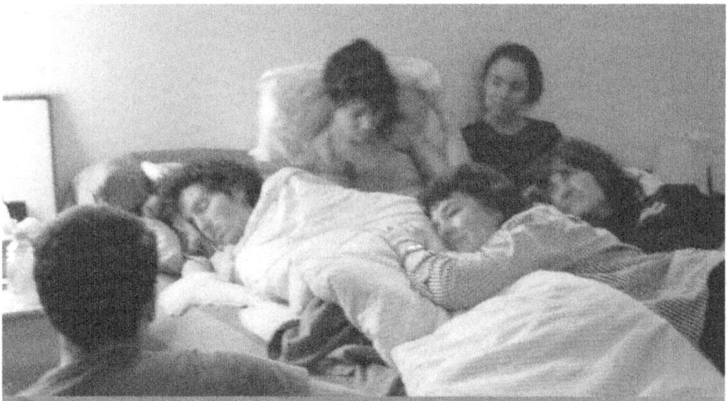

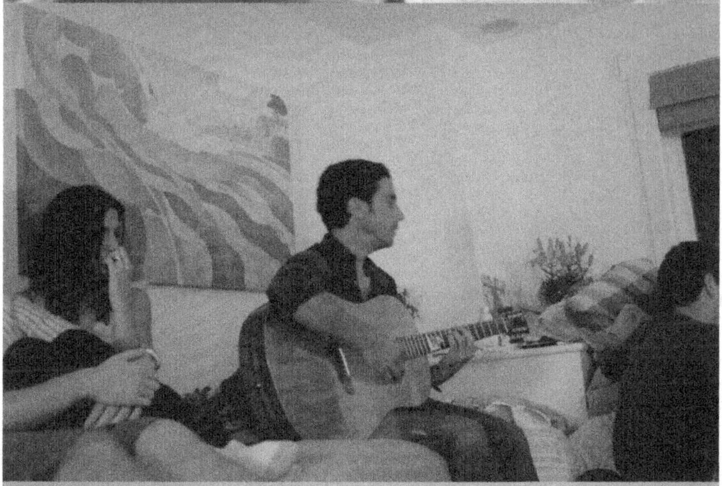

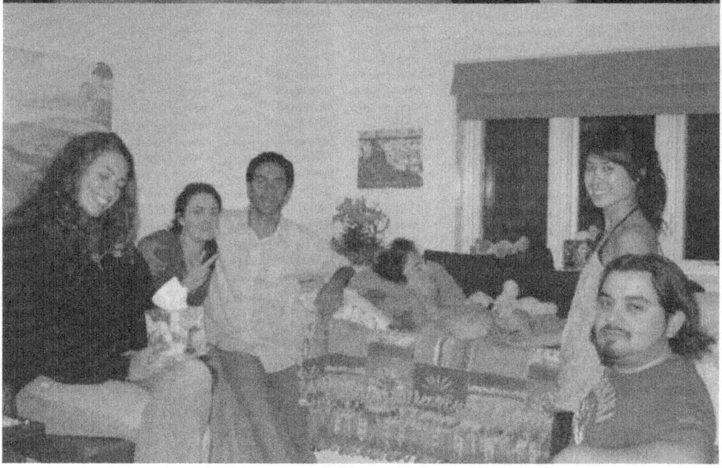

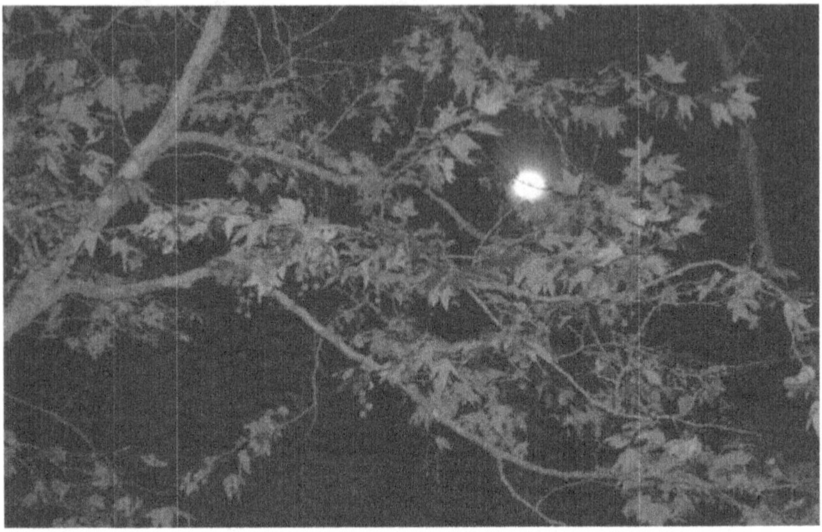

Danny died early in the morning on Halloween, 2007.

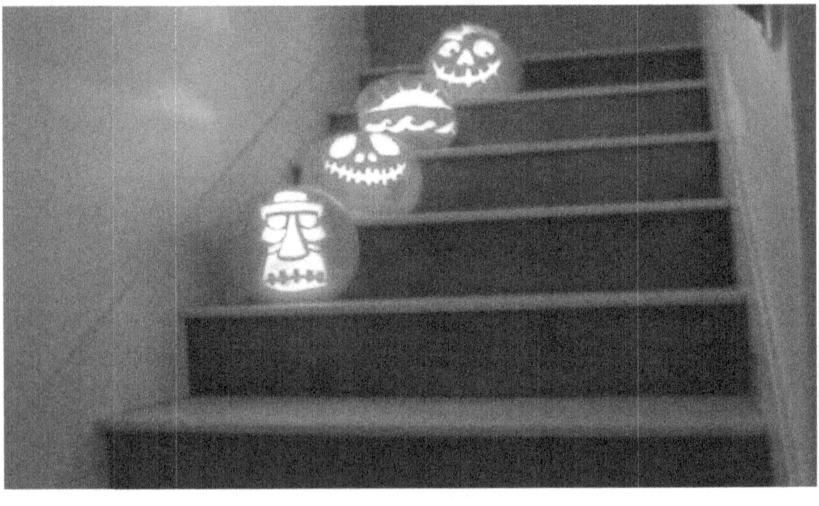

In the refection below, I tried to share the darkness and light of my son's death:

Soul-Son

The gift of a son is:
a treasure,
a trust,
a test,
a today,
a tomorrow,
and at times
a tragedy.

Loss of a son
is that tragic moment
of helplessness,
despair,
pain,
panic,
fear,
death of a young loved one
provokes.

Yet, my son lives on,
as we continue
in the loving relationship
of father and son.
He becomes my soul-son.
The son who lives, loves,
from within.

Danny lives
in the deepest part of me,
my soul.
He is my soul-son,
The gift
I cannot see,
but feel,
accompanying,
inspiring,
loving
his ever-grateful;
dad,
father,
poppy.

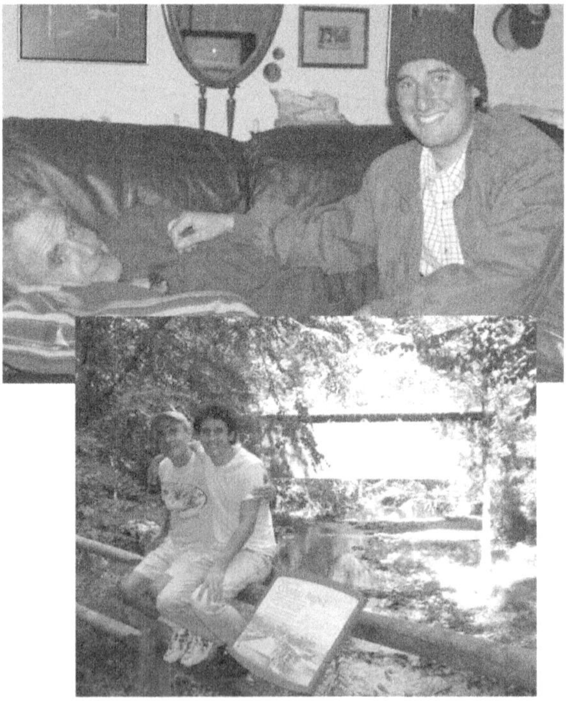

25
Beyond The Horizon

The silence of Danny's death was broken by activities to continue to share the gifts of his life, beginning with an almost immediate call for arrangements to donate his eyes so that others could see through them. Maggi, Alicia, and Catherine were interviewed for the articles in the San Diego Union-Tribune and UCSB school paper about Danny.

DAILY NEXUS
University of California, Santa Barbara

Published Monday, November 5, 2007 - Issue 30 / Volume 88 By Aria Miran / Staff Writer

Family, Friends To Memorialize Life of UCSB Student

Second-Year Danny Riley Dies From Rare Brain Tumor; Family Sets Up Fund

Catherine's quote in this article will always echo in my life: "Everyone hoped for a miracle. Danny is the miracle." The reporter also quoted Maggi extensively:

> Baker said her son liked to express himself by writing music and singing along to the guitar he taught himself to play in high school.

> 'That guitar and his own singing voice was where he sounded best,' Baker said. 'He had a gift. In his short life he wrote a lot of nice songs.'

Danny's songs have lyrics about his death, but he never really spoke about it, except early one morning in the summer of 2007 when I was by his bed in the hospital. When Danny woke up, he asked me if I wanted to be cremated when I die and I said yes and that I wanted him to make sure some of my ashes were spread on the East Coast (Ocean City, New Jersey) and some on the West because I have lived my life on both coasts. He replied sure he would take care of it. Then he said that he wanted to be cremated too and have his ashes spread in the sea but that he also wanted a memorial, not anything too religious but something living, so people could come and remember him.

After that early morning father-son chat, I have taken Danny's wishes to heart, which is probably why I am writing these words. I want a living memorial of Danny, our miracle, the singer, poet, and student of life, who became a teacher of how to live fully and die in peace, surrounded by circles of love.

Since it was clear that Danny wanted his body to be cremated, we arranged for that right away and then began plans for a Celebration of Life which many family and friends from near and far wanted to attend and did. One of our many projects was to make a bookmark with something about his life and a couple of his poems:

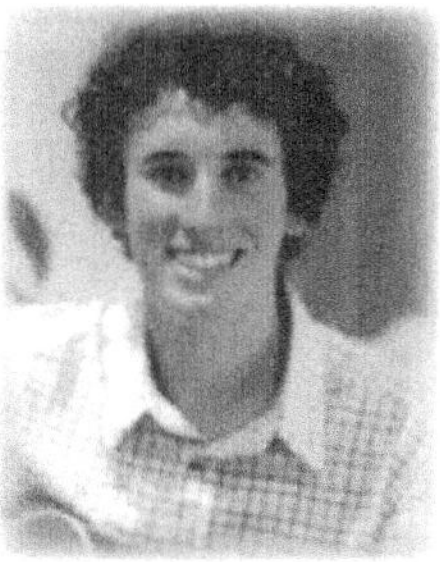

Daniel Joseph Riley
December 12, 1987 - October 31, 2007

If I could
I'd give every child
A terrestrial globe...
If possible, even
A globe that would light up,
In the hope
Of opening those young eyes
As wide as they will go
And arousing interest in,
and love for,
All peoples,
All races,
All tongues,
All religions!

—Dom Helder Camara
A Thousand Reasons for Living

Danny's birth announcement included this wish and his own poetry reflects it.

World of Love

Make me into a world of love
Passion in my soul
and kindness in my heart
Bend the skin which binds my cast
Heal me once and it will forever last.
Take me from the devil's rays
Hold me close for all my days
The sky is bright with tender hope
I feel it in the words Ive wrote
Simply am I on the path
Alone and blind I search and laugh
To find my peace that is my quest
To fulfill my life is my end at last.

-Danny Riley

Ivory Angel

im tired of all the killing
why cant we care for the poor?
with so much hatred and anger
we can all do a little more

come and kiss them ivory angel
they need to see your healing light
come and kiss them ivory angel
the last thing we need is
another fight

with all of us
bound together with our hearts
we can find the answers
to the questions that keep us apart

-Danny Riley

More of Danny's writings and music are available on his website: www.dannyriley.com

While the Celebration of Life was on Saturday evening, Joe and Posy Dibos had a festive celebration for family and friends at their house the night before. It was like an Irish wake but singing and laughter overshadowed any stories that might have been told. Joe had a large picture of Danny made and many smaller ones, as well as tee shirts with Danny's picture on them. It was a comforting reflection of the love and support for Danny and our family.

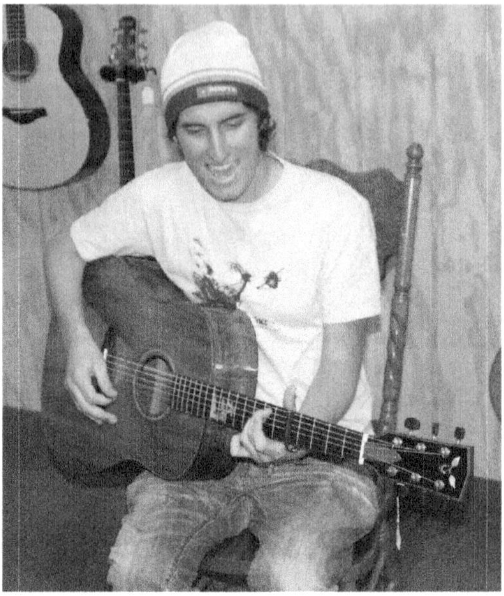

The next evening we had the Celebration of Life service at Saint Francis Chapel next to the Mission in San Diego. It was a Catholic Mass but threaded throughout were elements of other faiths, including the sermon delivered by the Rev. Madison Shockley, pastor of the Pilgrim United Church of Christ in Carlsbad, California, where the Rev. Gordon Baker, Danny's grandfather, was pastor emeritus and Maggi is a member. Madison knew Danny and had been with us in the hospital when bad news from a scan was shared. This was not a sermon given by a preacher who barely knew the deceased. Madison's words were from the heart of a gifted man of faith who loved Danny, laughed with him and cried with us. I can still hear his eloquent words: Danny did not choose to go to the Great Wall of China, or visit some exotic land. He wanted to stay with those he loved and who loved him because that was where his life was. He chose to live here with us. And how he lived! He sang, wrote, laughed, and loved! He lived and kept on living fully until his final breath.

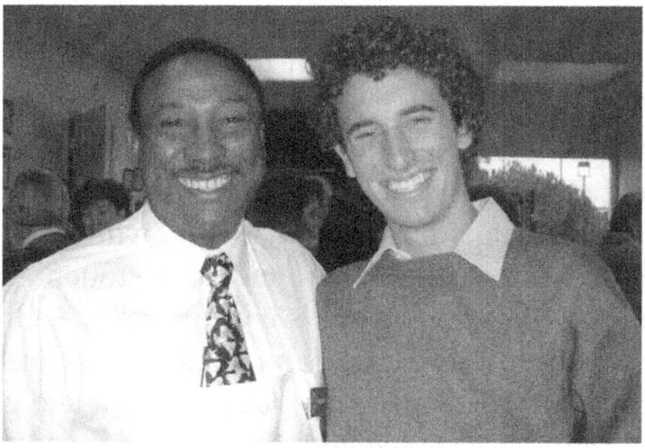

Rev. Madison Shockley and Danny

Madison's words were soon followed by prayers of the faithful, the Catholic petition prayers, which were voiced by family and friends. We crafted them to include the hopes for the causes Danny espoused, hope for cures for persons like Danny, acknowledgement of those who cared for him and continue to care for others. Beyond the ritual of the Mass itself, the symbolic highlight may have been the Offertory procession, which is when the main elements of the Mass, the bread and wine, are brought up. We took this as an opportunity to bring the gifts of Danny's life: his guitar, demo CD, saxophone, skateboard, all-star soccer jacket, ASB jacket, basketball, the banner of love that was made for his hospital room, the Word board, flowers carried by Alicia and Catherine, and finally a large picture that remained in the center for the rest of the service. While there were tears throughout, the final part when everyone was given a candle, the lights dimmed, and we had the song "Wanting Memories" by the Stanford accapella group, Talisman, followed by Danny's recording of Ben Harper's "Waiting on an Angel" were the real "tear jerkers."

Tears turned to a joyful celebration in the California Room below the chapel, which was filled with pictures of Danny throughout his life, with his music playing in the background, and a touching slide show done by, Danny's cousin, Jacob Tell. This was followed by songs by Danny's cousins Ashley and Michael Arnold, Jack Johnson and good friend Mathew MacAvene. I felt that the room was alive in celebration of Danny's life.

The next memorable event was the paddle out. Since Danny loved the ocean and was an occasional surfer, a paddle out to spread his ashes was appropriate. Danny's cousin Kim and her husband Jack took the lead in helping us arrange it for the Saturday after Thanksgiving at their house in Santa Barbara, where Danny died.

Words can't describe the paddle out but some pictures of the circle of love on the beach and the smaller circle of those who went into the water may. Whatever one believes about death, the life of the sea and the love of the person whose ashes go to it fill you with a deep respect for the cycle of life and our own connection to nature and each other.

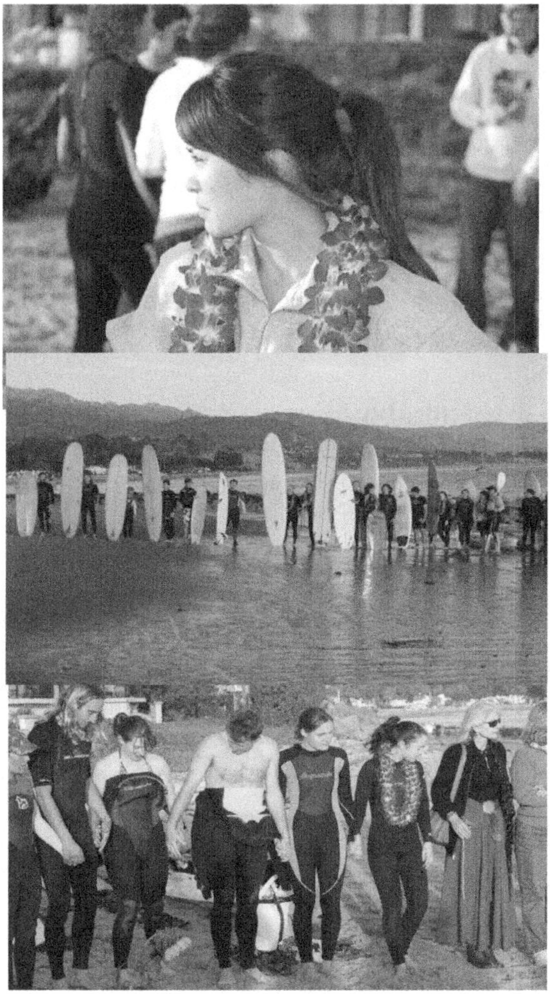

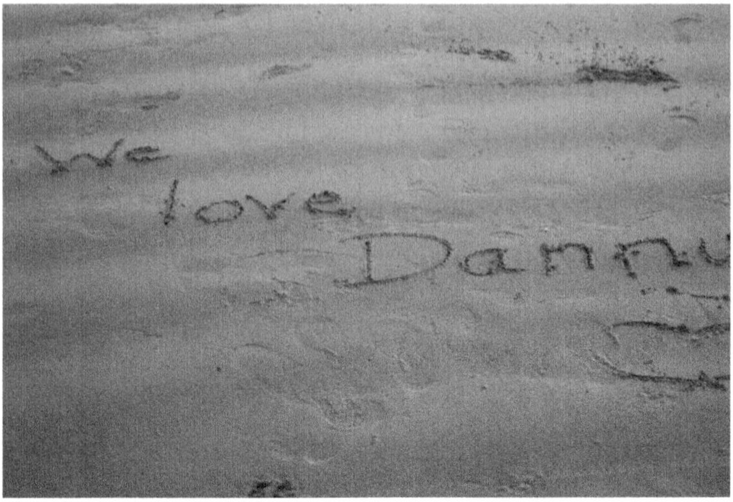

In this reflection, I try to express what missing a loved one may mean:

Missing Danny

The sun that has just set brings an afterglow,
a rap of bright colors.
I don't miss the sun because it will shine
again when the new day dawns.

Danny's smile set behind the horizon of
death, leaving memories of his laugh, and
love.
I miss that smile because there will be no
new day to see it shine.

The missing penetrates every day and draws a yearning for a new way to feel his presence.

The missing is a catalyst, an angst, a longing for a new feeling of Danny.

The missing began as sadness and it still colors it, but it's a positive feeling too.

Missing Danny means seeking his sense of wonder, music, and closeness.

Missing Danny means not wanting to lose his magic, his glow, his call to feel, and listen to life's magic.

Missing is a way of connecting, calling out for an ongoing relationship that crosses the horizons life brings, even the one death presents.

Missing is memory, but more: meaning, moments of the heart. It is magic because it defies eye's clear view to allow for a sense of wonder.

Missing is wondering how to live in the void that death brings. Yet, is an opening to how to bridge it, to connect to the soul's new relationship with the spirit of a wonderful son.

Missing is a vacillating feeling because Danny is not fully gone.

While I miss seeing his smile, feeling his touch, hearing is voice, I can't miss all of him because he is still present in my deepest feelings.

I will not always miss Danny because the missing will fade as I listen to his call to reach inward, to be with him, to sing his new song, to let his new life always be a part of mine.

26
Unfinished Books

Danny was a reader, which is probably why he was also a writer of songs, poems, and the beginning of his own story. We still have not changed Danny's room, mainly because the walls have writings that were inspirational quotes and reminders to live each day to its fullest.

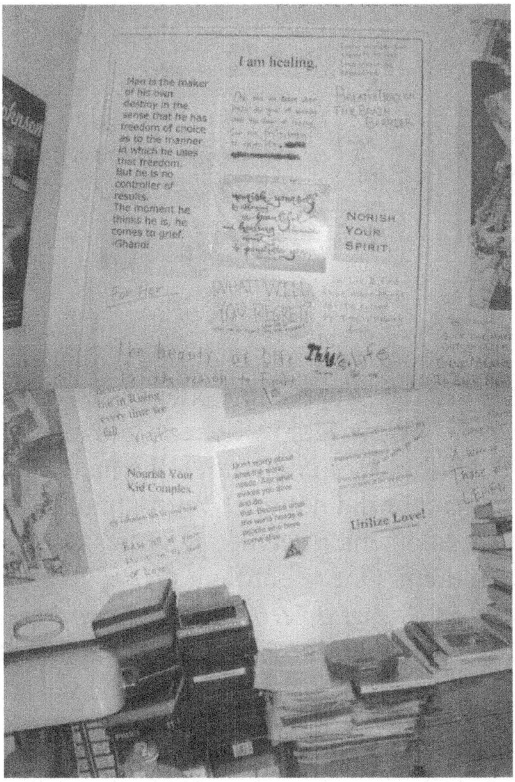

On his bed board, he wrote the famous line from *Dead Poets Society*: "Carpe Diem," seize the day, which Danny certainly tried to do and did, despite the progression of his cancer.

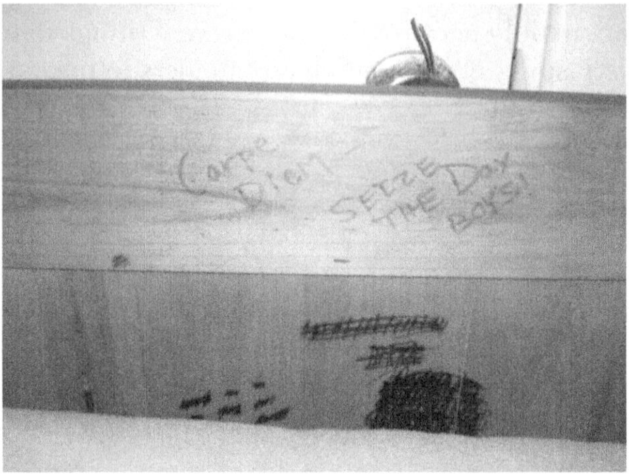

In Danny's room there are books of philosophy, poetry, mysteries, the Harry Potter series, and many about music. While I know he read and re-read the Harry Potter books, I could not tell which of his books he read or did not read, but I noticed two that had bookmarks which seemed to indicate how far he read in them. One is entitled: *OUR APPOINTMENT with LIFE: Discourse on Living Happily in the Present Moment,* by Thich Nhat Hanh. While it is a short book about the wisdom of Buddhism, the bookmark was between pages six and seven. Now that might have been far enough for Danny because page five contains the following words:

> Do not pursue the past
> Do not lose yourself in the future.
> The past no longer is.
> The future has not yet come.
> Looking deeply at life as it is
> in the very here and now,
> the practitioner dwells
> in stability and freedom.
> We must be diligent today.
> To wait until tomorrow is too late.
> Death comes unexpectedly.
> How can we bargain with it?
> The sage calls a person who knows
> How to dwell in mindfulness
> Night and day…

Danny lived these words and often commented that he did not want to know where his brain cancer came from, what caused it, or where it was going, but how to live a normal life with it now, which he did.

Another unfinished book is *The Reasons of Love* by Harry G. Frankfurt. This is a short book about philosophy. The bookmark is between pages 20 and 21. On page 14 are these words:

> In managing and designing their lives,
> people need to confront a number
> of significant issues. They must make up
> their minds concerning what

> they want, which things they want more than
> others, what they consider to
> be intrinsically valuable and hence
> appropriate for pursuit not just as
> a means but as a final end, and what they in
> fact will pursue as final ends.
> In addition, they face a distinct further task.
> They have to determine what it is they care
> about.

Another book I found in Danny's room contains pencil marks to highlight phrases that caught his attention. Tim O'Brien's award-winning novel about soldiers in the Vietnam War, entitled: *The Things They Carried* has a bookmark between pages 82 and 83. Danny underlined parts of pages 81 and 82 and put stars next to two sections which tell about how living in the face of death brings a deeper appreciation of life. Rather than quote these, I copied them to give a sense of Danny reading, underlining, and marking them with stars showing what they meant to him, that he would face death by being positive, caring, kind, and appreciative of the gifts of each day.

...

proximity to death brings with it a corresponding proximity to life. After a firefight, there is always the immense pleasure of aliveness. The trees are alive. The grass, the soil—everything. All around you things are purely living, and you among them, and the aliveness makes you tremble. You feel an intense, out-of-the-skin awareness of your living self—your truest self, the human being you want to be and then become by the force of wanting it. In the midst of evil you want to be a good man. You want decency. You want justice and courtesy and human concord, things you never knew you wanted. There is a kind of largeness to it, a kind of godliness. Though it's odd, you're never more alive than when you're almost dead. You recognize what's valuable. Freshly, as if for the first time, you love what's best in yourself and in the world, all that might be lost.

Page 81

...

you find yourself studying the fine colors on the river, you feel wonder and awe at the setting of the sun, and you are filled with a hard, aching love for how the world could be and always should be, but now is not.

Page 82

Well, Danny certainly determined what he cared about: the people he loved and those who loved him, music, living fully each day in a positive way and helping others smile at cancer as he did, "beating it with love," to use his expression.

This book about Danny's story will always be unfinished because Danny's almost twenty years left the lyrics of his life, melodies, and wonder at what might have been. In a sense, Danny's journey continues in the lives of those who knew him and others who have learned about him. It resonates in the deepest yearnings of all of us who face the challenges of each day, to live them with courage, care, and concern for others.

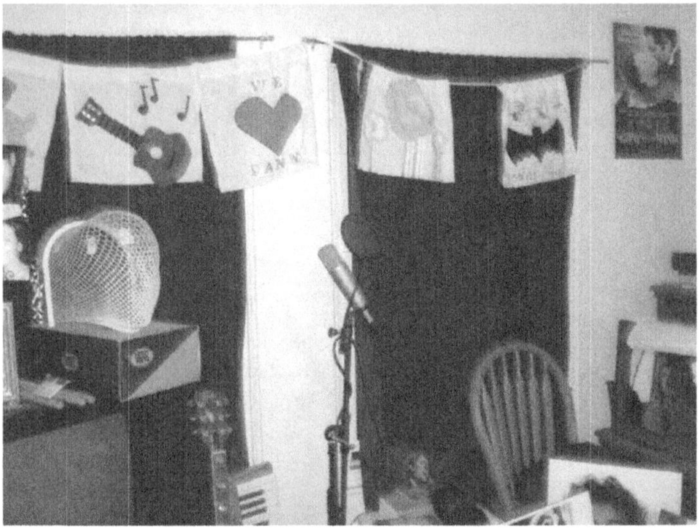

27
The Ginkgo Trees

Earlier I wrote that Danny wanted something living as a memorial, so people could come to remember him. One of his poems concluded with this refrain:

dont you know me?
dont you know me by now?
someday we'll see.
someday we'll see.
dont forget about me.
dont forget about me.
--"A Prayer" by Danny

Danny wrote another poem about a tree:

Shade From the Gold Tree

giving my heart
shouting your name
tripping on roots
as i walk through your forest.

i come to your tree
with leaves of gold
and bark of diamond
it is all alone.
through the leaves the sun shines
blinding my fixed eyes
the light's so pure it makes me cry
i turn back and stumble home.

when im back i can only think
of that tree in the forest
if only i could have found its shade.

that night i went back
crept through the woods
like a nimble cat

until i reached the same gold tree
i touched the bark but it felt cold to me
reflecting off the leaves the moon did shine
brighter than ever, burning my eyes.

i took a step back
regained my sense
stood mesmorized by the gold light
lost my will to fight

that night i dreamt
of sitting beneath the tree
and catching its leaves
as they fell down to me.

and when i woke i was there in the shade
the light did shine
but the shade did impair
its harm.

So it seemed right that one of the places of

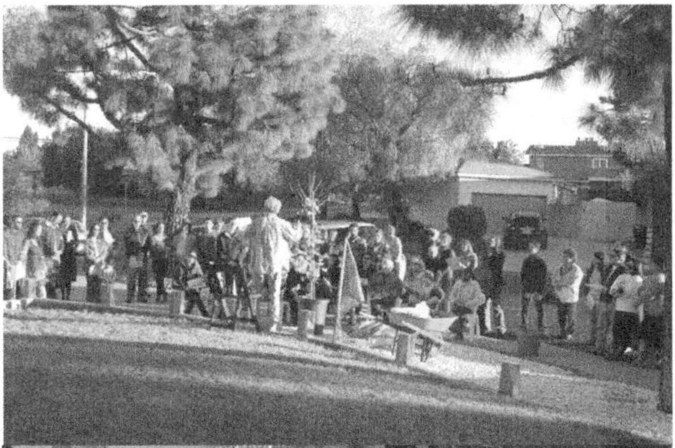

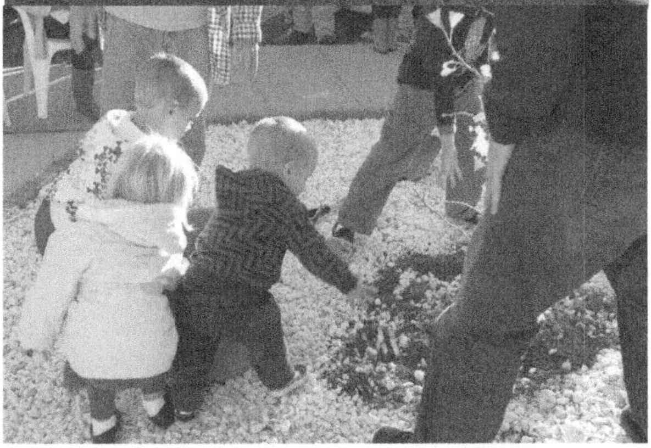

rememberance would be a tree planted at our home in Chula Vista, where Danny grew up. After Christmas of 2008, family and friends gathered for the planting of a gingko tree. We found a recording by Danny reciting the poem above and played it as we planted the tree as a symbol of his life and our continuing connection to it. Just as their parents had surrounded Danny in his short life, the littlest cousins put the dirt around his tree.

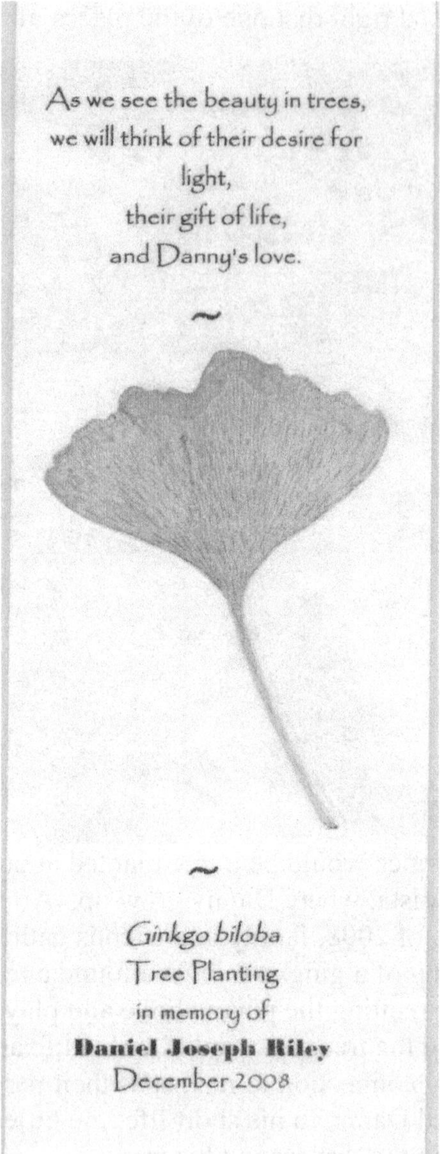

Bookmark made for the occasion

Another ginkgo tree was planted for Danny in the patio at the UCSB Student Health Center by Dr. Elizabeth Downing and her dedicated staff.

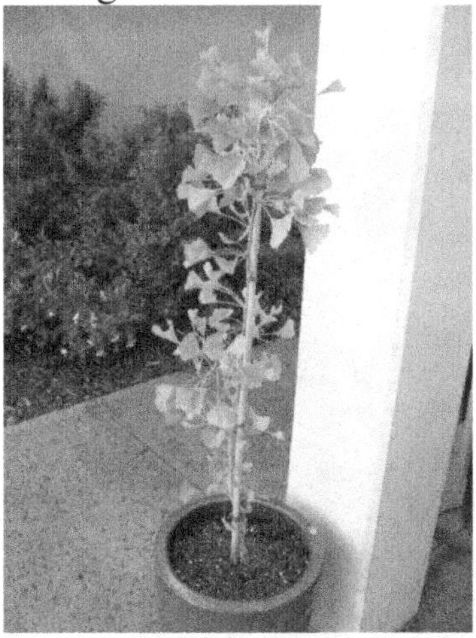

Next to the tree we placed a rock engaved with the follwing message:

Danny Riley ~ Class of 2010
December 12, 1987 - October 31, 2007

Despite being diagnosed with brain cancer during high school, Danny fulfilled his dream to attend UCSB and live life to the fullest. Here he found support and friendships that helped him to thrive as long as possible. Through his songs and poetry, we continue to feel Danny's wisdom, love, and positive spirit.

28
Hope

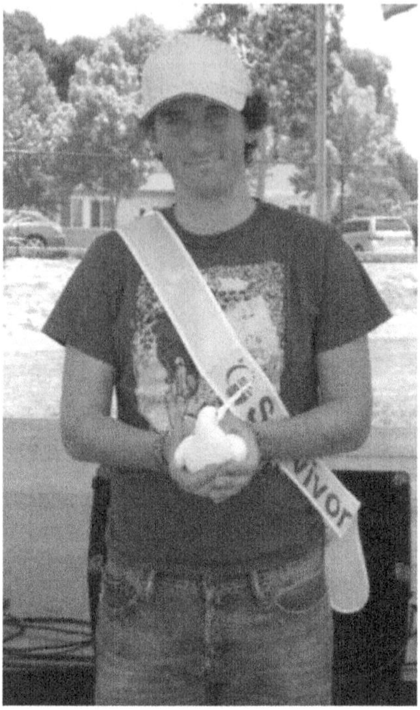

This picture shows what hope looked like in the summer of 2006. Danny took part in a clinical trial that gave him a terrible rash but also hope that it would be the breakthrough drug that could cure his cancer and make him a long-time survivor. All of us need hope but those with cancer need it in their core. Danny lost his battle with cancer but he never lost hope that he could live a full life with it. He said he would undergo any treatment, take any chemo available, and was open to any clinical trial.

Earlier I referred to his answers to an applicaton for a scholarhsip from the Pedicatic Brain Tumor Foundation. In response to a question about what advice would you give someone who just found out he or she had a brain tumor, Danny wrote: "Beat it with love." In a sense, Danny beat his own tumor. While cancer took his life, it never drained him of love nor hope. On the contrary, it seemed to make him more aware of love and hope and a desire to share these gifts with others. He wanted to live fully despite his disease, and as he wrote, even embrace it. Danny's story is about that hope. His journey continues in our hopes for a cure, our commitment to the causes that fight for this goal, and our caring for the survivors of any length of time who teach us the beauty of life's "now."

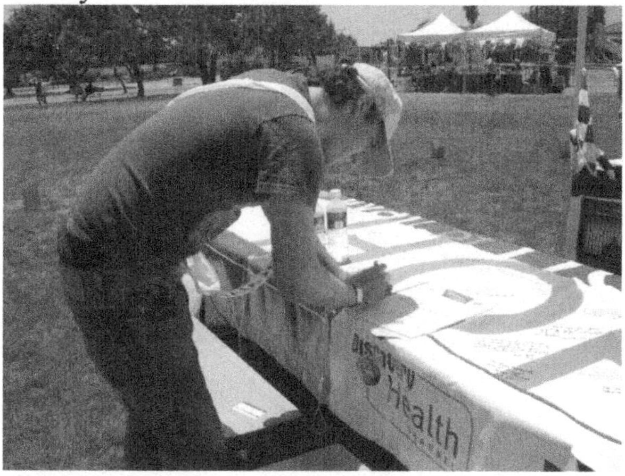

Beyond the horizon there will always be the the light of a new day, a dawn that will brighten those like Danny with news that will reward and honor their hope for a cure. Danny's story, his poetry, and songs continue to reflect such a hope.

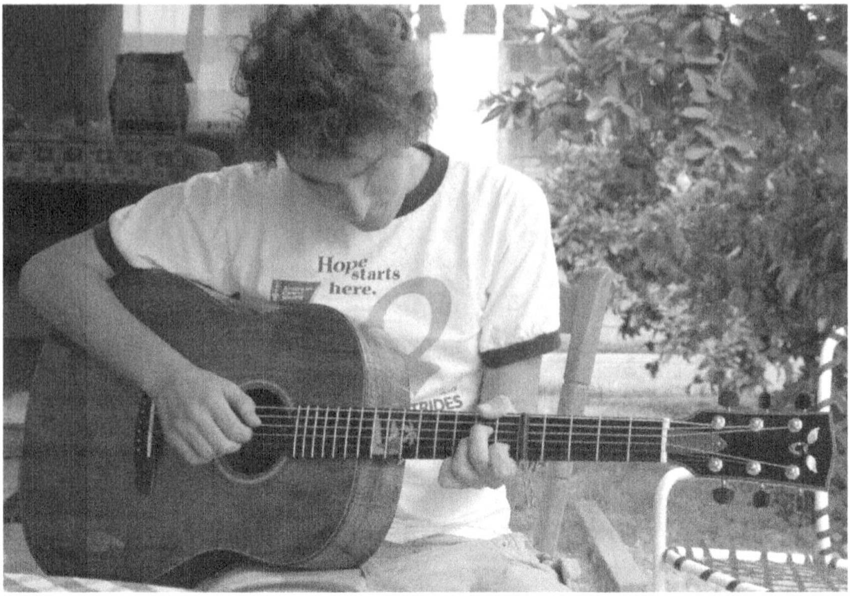

"The sky is bright with tender hope!"
-Danny

29
Projects and Thanks

Many years ago, I read a novel by William Saroyan, entitled: ***The Human Comedy***. In it there are words about pain that I will always remember:

> If a man has not wept at the world's pain he is only half a man, and there will always be pain in the world. Knowing this does not mean that a man shall despair. A good man will seek to take pain out of things.

Before December 8, 2004, I thought I had wept at the world's pain and what had touched me: the deaths of my parents (in my early 30s), of my brother Bill (the year Danny was born), and of other close family and friends. But the pain that touched my life beginning December 2004 and reached its peak on October 31, 2007, cut to the core of my limits. Life's wonder is that we can handle it. I feel the fullness of life is still with us in the gifts of the human spirit, touched by grace. I see life's wonder manifested in the love of family, friends, and fellow travelers on life's journey. I think Danny knew this, experienced it, shared it, and still does. As Danny wrote, he would embrace pain if he could only keep his love. In embracing the pain of Danny's life and death, I feel his life, love, and light (Danny's mantra) stronger. My hope is that the gifts of Danny's life and journey can be shared.

This sharing started shortly before the memorial service with the thoughtful action of Debbie Bosetti, who is the mother of Danny's good friend Mike Bosetti and in 2007 was a staff member at Family House, where we stayed when Danny was being treated at UCSF Medical Center in San Francisco. Debbie offered to set up a Danny Riley Celebration of Life Fund so there would be place for family and friends to give donations at the service and afterwards.

When it became more efficient to manage the funds from San Diego, we moved the fund to the Danny Riley Celebration of Life Fund at The San Diego Foundation. We also left some of the original donations at Family House to help children staying there during their medal care to experience the healing power of music.

In San Diego we have partnered with a nonprofit organization A Reason To Survive (ARTS) which honored Danny's memory by establishing the "Danny Riley Music Program." Here are more details about the fund and the music program at ARTS:

> As a tribute to Danny, his friends and family set up **The Danny Riley Celebration of Life Fund** to help children and young adults with cancer and other serious conditions to experience the healing art of music.

For ten years, The Danny Riley Celebration of Life Fund was administered by The San Diego Foundation. And during that time over $40,000 in donations were given to non-profits in Danny's name. However, we closed it in 2018. We continue to support the Danny Riley Music Program at ARTS, which is a San Diego non-profit organization that is dedicated to healing, inspiring, and empowering children facing life challenges by providing innovative arts-based programs, education, and opportunities. ARTS provides various opportunities for children to express themselves through various art mediums, such as visual arts, media art, and music, as they face life challenges ranging from having a disease to living in poverty. More information on ARTS can be found at their website: www.areasontosurvive.org.

The sharing continued when Jack and Kim Johnson set up the Danny Riley Fund, described in this Press Release, at UCSB:

UCSB Alumnus and Songwriter Jack Johnson Donates $50,000 for Disabled Students January 26, 2010
(Santa Barbara, Calif.) — Singer and songwriter Jack Johnson and his wife, Kim, both UC Santa Barbara graduates, have

made a $50,000 contribution to the campus to support students with serious medical conditions through the Disabled Students Program. The recent gift honors the courageous life of Danny Riley, who was a UCSB student when he died of brain cancer in 2007.

The Danny Riley Fund will help undergraduates with cancer and other serious illnesses to pursue their education at UCSB by providing support for financial aid, medication, housing, adaptive equipment, home care, transportation, family visits, and other special needs.

"Our cousin, Danny Riley, lived life to the fullest and didn't let his battle with cancer deter him from his dream of attending UCSB," said Jack Johnson. "Kim and I created the Danny Riley Fund to support students who face similar challenges and to pass along Danny's zest for life."

Gary White, director of the campus's Disabled Students Program, expressed his sincere gratitude to the Johnsons for their important contribution. "The Danny Riley Fund is already helping students by making it possible for parents to be here at critical times," he said. "This very generous gift will greatly enhance the services we provide."

Riley, Kim Johnson's cousin, was diagnosed with brain cancer in his junior year of high school. He wrote about the experience on his application to UCSB, noting that "living a

> normal life with cancer" was one of his "proudest achievements." Despite interruptions for medical treatment, he was an honor student at UCSB. Riley shared Jack Johnson's passion for music and sang background vocals on one of his recordings. "Danny said he was always meeting angels at UCSB in the disabled students office and at the health center, angels who helped him in every way they could," said his father, Frank Riley. Last fall, the Riley family hosted a reception on campus to thank those who knew and supported their son. A tree was planted in Danny Riley's memory in the patio of the Student Health Services building.

While the initial funding has been used, this fund continues and we hope to keep it going into the future.

Danny's cousin Jacob Tell has initiated several projects which share Danny with others. He set up a website (www.dannyriley.com) and is helping us reformat and develop an expanded design. Through his company Oniric Records, Jacob also produced *Solutions for Dreamers* albums 1, 2 and 3, each of which includes one of Danny's songs. He also has plans for a tribute album with artists covering Danny's songs.

We compiled Danny's original songs in a special album *Conversation (take two)*, which includes photos and lyrics.

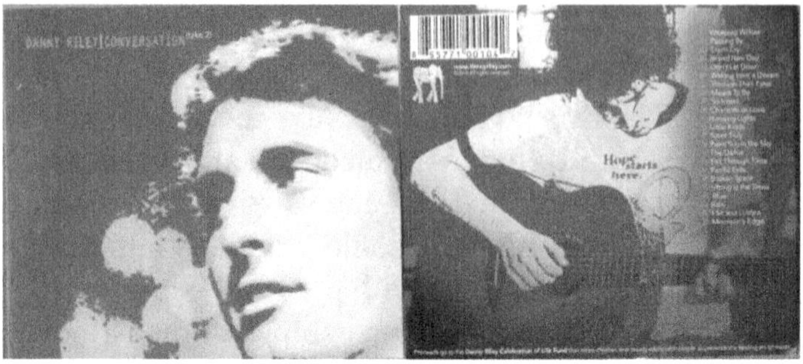

We just finished another album, *Going Home* with four covers including Danny's touching version of Dolly Parton's *I Will Always Love You,* which we discovered on his computer after his death. These are combined with four of Danny's original songs.

Another project is this book, which I hope will bring people to know Danny a support our efforts in his name.

An ongoing "labor of love" is expressing appreciation to all those who shared Danny's journey, especially: Catherine Omalev, her parents, brother, aunts and spouses. Our deep appreciation also goes to: the Bosetti family, especially Mike Bosetti, all Danny's friends at UCSB, Gary White and the staff at the Student Disability Center at UCSB, the staff at Family House in San Francisco, the teachers, counselors, and fellow students at

Eastlake High School who supported Danny in his journey and so many others along the way.

Maggi received important information and support for her role as Danny's caregiver through participation in the San Diego Brain Tumor Support Group.

We will always be grateful to Doctors Banerjee, and Gupta, Nurse Practitioner Caroline Pearson and to the rest of caring staff at UCSF Medical Center and Hospital, as well as the members of the Brain Tumor Board.

Dr. McQuaide at Kaiser Permanente was Danny's pediatrician for most of his life and by his side for major events during his battle with cancer. Special thanks go to him, and all the physicians and staff at Kaiser in San Diego and Los Angeles.

Previously I mentioned Dr. Downing and her caring staff at the UCSB Health Center, as well as the wonderful staff of the Cancer Center of Santa Barbara and Cottage Hospital. In the summer of 2007, Danny was a frequent patient at the Cancer Center of San Diego, where he met Dr. Paul Brenner, a caring physician and psychologist who went out of his way to be with Danny, even visiting him in Santa Barbara.

There were many nurses, medical technicians, and attendants who came in and out of Danny's life who tried as hard as they could to help Danny but special note has to be made of Jack Lowry, the nurse in Dr. McQuaide's office and Dawn Robertson who facilitated getting the many MRI reports at Kaiser in San Diego.

While having a young loved one in hospice care was painful, Susanna Dubler and Barbara Pell of Visiting Nurse & Hospice Care of Santa Barbara were gentle caregivers to Danny and our family.

One of our special friends is Jim Murray, former General Manager of the Philadelphia Eagles and one of the founders of the Ronald MacDonald Houses. Jim got a copy of Danny's college application essay and was so touched by it that he uses it in his speeches to inspire others. He contacted a foundation to help cover some of the expenses for Danny's treatment and care. His many calls and Irish Blessings were wonderful touches to our lives in a very difficult time.

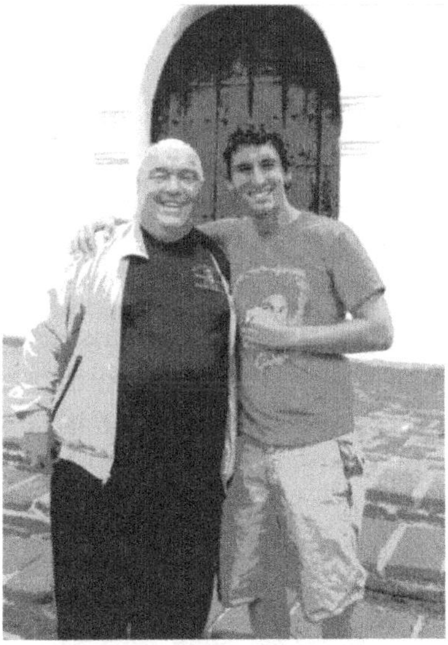

Jim Murray and Danny

We had financial help along the way from individuals and groups. There were three informal Danny funds: one from the extended Riley Clan, another from the extended Dibos family, and Joe Dibos called upon former Augustinians to help. While we had health insurance, there were many expenses that these funds helped us meet so we could provide Danny with the best of care.

We are especially grateful for the ongoing sharing of music. We have tried to listen to it in the way Danny did to feel the life, love, and light from the lyrics, melodies, and magic moments it creates. Many helped Danny enjoy this gift in his life, especially Matt MacAvene, Anders Bergstrom, and other members of Matt's band that Danny jammed with and even performed with at Rocks as well as at the Heal the Ocean concert in Santa Barbara.

We are so grateful for the love and support that Jack Johnson gave to Danny even before he married Kim. Danny looked up to Jack as a role model and big brother. Jack gave Danny tips on his music, even helped him record one of his songs "Passing By" at his studio in Hawaii. Jack also made sure that Danny sang back-up vocals on the song "If I Had Eyes," which they recorded at Jack's studio in Los Angeles in September 21, 2007. After Danny died, we were stunned by the beauty of the ***Sleep through the Static*** album cover and dedication of the album to Danny's memory.

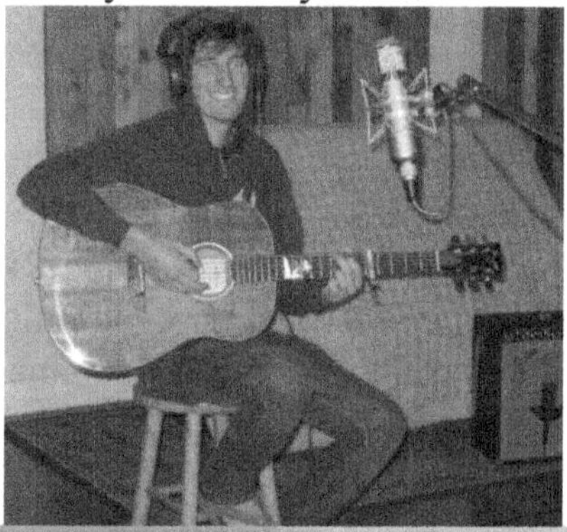

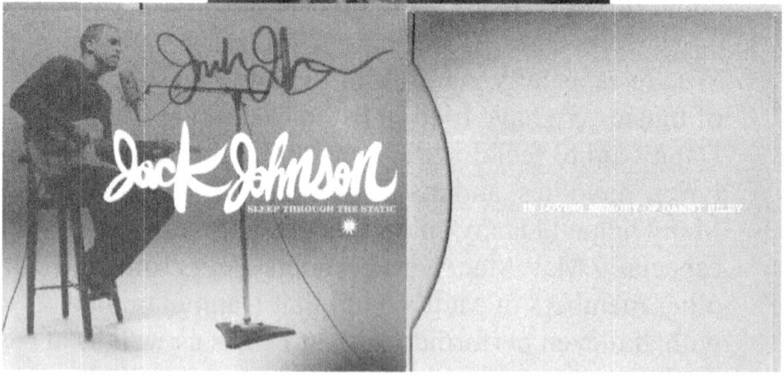

A month after Danny died, Jack asked if he could borrow the Goodall Koa guitar (in the picture above) that was given to Danny in August 2007. He didn't tell us why at the time, but we later saw it on stage in a video of one of his shows on the **Sleep through the Static** concert tour. Jack and his crew placed it on stage at his shows all over the world and brought it back to us at his concert in Chula Vista 2008. Jack also dedicated a song "Go On" to Danny and spoke about his guitar coming home.

Well, it did not stay home long. We came to know and love a gifted singer/songwriter, Michael Tiernan, a cancer survivor. He is a kindred spirit because he is former seminarian who studied in Rome, which I did in 1966-1968. I felt an immediate connection to him and his music, which is laced with lyrics and melodies that lift the spirit.

We went to some of Michael's gigs and learned that he was recording a new album, so we asked if he would like to use Danny's Koa guitar for it and he said yes. The new album: "LA Can Wait" was released on September 15, 2010 and the cover mentions Danny's guitar. The songs are great, especially "Strong" which is about his own brother Joe's battle with cancer (**www.Tiernantunes.com**).

Through Jack's website, we have come to know other families who lost children to cancer, like the

McDonalds in England. Their son Sam was another budding singer who died at age 17.

When I wrote the first edition of this book (2011) we still had not met them but have corresponded, exchanging stories and projects about our sons, including the CD "Play It Again Sam"

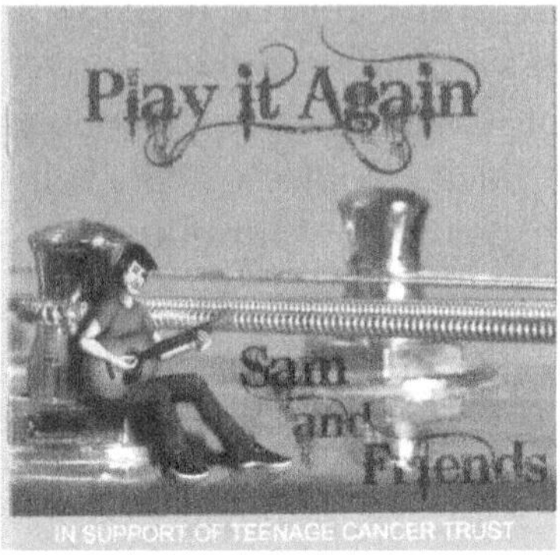

that they and their son's friends made to raise funds for a TEENAGE CANCER TRUST in England (www.teenagecancertrust.org). Then, in June of 2015, Kevin and Jane McDonald came for a visit to the U.S. which included staying a few wonderful days with us. On the night before they left, Jane gave us a poem she wrote about our two sons, entitled "Our Boys":

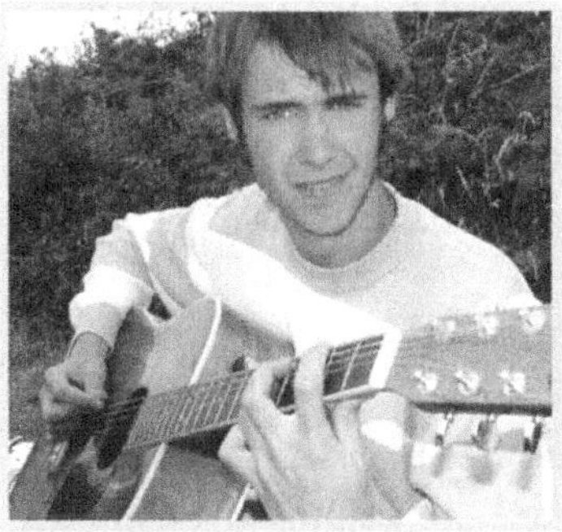

Sam McDonald

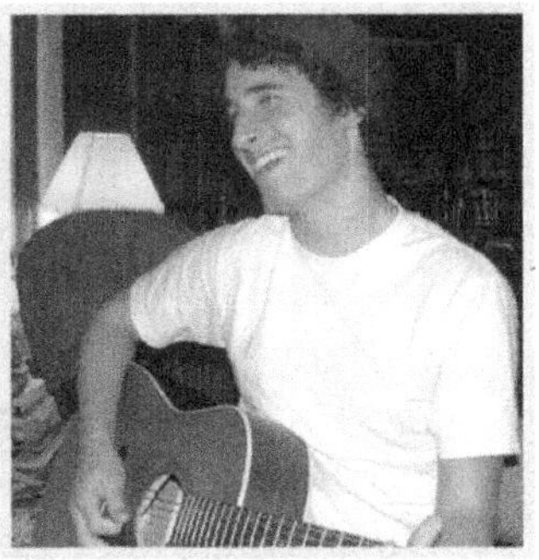

Danny Riley

<u>Our Boys</u>

Danny and Sam lived worlds apart
But both had music and words in their heart
Working hard and having fun
Chilling out in rain or sun

But their bodies were thinking a different way
As they were told on that fateful day
December the 8th 2004
Changed our lives for evermore

Tests then followed, with biopsies and scans
Results, discussions and treatment plans
Side effects, transfusions and infections were rife
As they both bravely continued on with their life

Loyalty reigned and friendships grew
With some not knowing what to do
Normality is what our boys desired
Though sometimes their bodies were just too tired

Hair fell out, but their smiles remained
As the roller coaster ride took its strain
Good news and bad came interspersed
Joy and tears were well rehearsed

Remission for a while we're full of joy
But it was just waiting to redeploy
The cancer returned and took its grip
Ding Ding, there started the round two trip
More plans and discussions with the team
And another grueling treatment regime
Pump in the poison and fire the rays
Keep positive amidst the fog and daze

Christmas and birthdays we celebrate
With uncertainty looming over future dates
Gathering around our family and friends
Appreciating the love and warmth it sends

The cancer's still there, but seems at bay
Maintenance is now the only way
Their bodies were tired, the road was tough
All in all they'd had enough

Acceptance was hard as everyone's told
There is no more, you're at the end of the road
Chats and hugs allaying fears
Trying to smile amidst the tears

Music helps soothe Sam's final days Jack Johnson
and Bob Marley float through the haze
Ethereal Sigur Ros and Damien Rice we play
All being grateful for another day

The June sun sees Sam breathe his last
The pain and suffering now in the past
Our hearts are broken but we try to be strong
To be angry or bitter would be so wrong

August sees Danny have another op
To keep it at bay there's no time to stop
In and out of Uni, keeping a routine
To those looking on, just a normal scene

In mid-October we head off to London
At Radio 2's Studios we see Jack Johnson
We're unaware of his thoughts on that day
As across the ocean Danny was slipping away

Two weeks later the fight is lost
Danny's battle is over at such a cost
More hearts broken, more empty lives
Faith and memories help you to survive

Mothers Day's hard, but Ross looks out for me
Giving me Jack's 'Sleep Through the Static'
music CD "In loving memory of Danny Riley"
I spied and after an e-mail or two our
families are tied

Our boys were so similar and so strong
What on earth caused it all to go so wrong?
Support we share with poetry and song
As the grieving path we all tread along

Tickets for Jack in Cornwall you sent
The weather was rough and wouldn't relent
Waterproofs on we all went with the flow
Singing along with Danny's guitar on show

Time goes on, yet seems to stand still
Each morning having to swallow that bitter pill
But we smile and know that our boys are fine
Singing and rocking in a land divine

Music helped their journeys along
Whether a heavy tune or a joyful song
'The Danny Riley Fund' you set up for your son
So others suffering could escape and have fun

While we chose to support 'Teenage Cancer Trust'
To improve the cancer journey had to be a must
Sam's dream was to provide appropriate care
So young people with cancer could chat and share

On different latitudes our grief's the same
Losing our sons brings such pain
But as the earth rotates through day and night
We cling to love with all our might

Eight years on and we meet at last

Looking to the future and talking of the past
Sharing our stories, our music and love
Listening for "Hallelujah's" floating above

-Jane McDonald

As I mentioned above, the McDonalds raised funds for the TEENAGE CANCER TRUST in England, which was founded by the surviving members of The WHO, rock stars Roger Daltry and Peter Townsend. They also shared that because of the TRUST's success in England, Daltry and Townsend founded a United States version of it called TEEN CANCER AMERCIA,www.teencanceramerica.org. After meeting meet several times with Executive Director, Simon Davies, and his team at their office in Los Angeles, we decided that along with other families to start of music program, based on what we experience with how music helped Danny. We hope this will help teenagers and young adults with cancer through music therapy and other music-related assistance as they travel on this hard journey. This program finally got up and running in 2018 and is called. Play It Back. Here's the link to it: https://teencanceramerica.org/news-resources/news/play-it-back-launch/

As I wrote earlier, my goal is to continue to share Danny's gifts. Along with Maggi, Alicia, and other family and friends, I want to remember Danny by helping others with challenges similar to his to experience the healing and hope that music can bring. Most of all, I want to share our family's gratitude for the gifts that are threaded throughout this story.

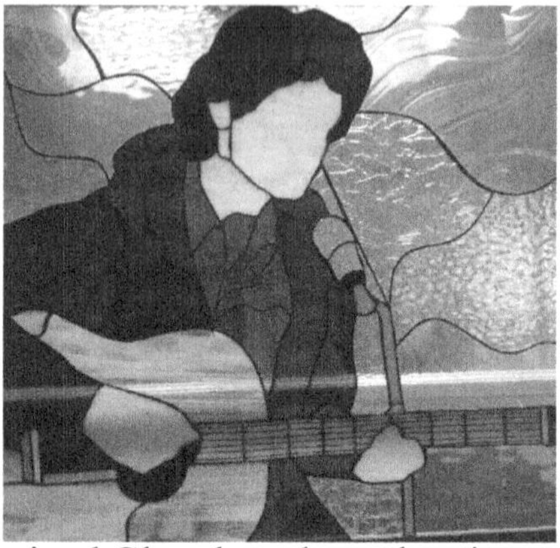

Stained Glass based on the picture of Danny below:

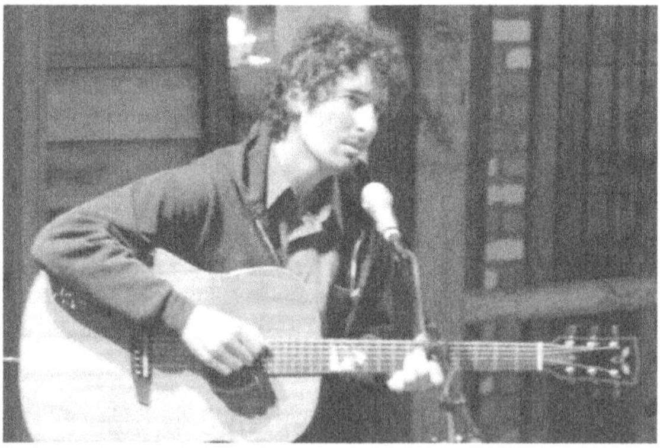

30
Left To Do

Danny wrote about the future in the following poem and wish, referenced in the Class of 2010 reflection:

what would a boy do if he knew
everything there was to know?
would he change the earth
or refuse to grow?
would he travel the world to meet new
friends?
or throw in his cards and wait for the end?
love and cherish all mankind?
wait and pray for an easier time?
it wouldnt be me
and it wouldnt be you
there is far too much
we have left to do.

◆◆◆◆◆

Live a life that is hard working
And true to yourself
Seek that which you desire;
Offer that which life inspires.
Recognize the beauty of life
And repay this gift,
Through the care you take in living well.
Then, life will repay you
for the services you've granted it.

There is "far too much we have left to do," but we can shine light in darkness, bring hope in despair, and joy in the midst of pain, especially if we "recognize the beauty of life and repay this gift."

31
Forever Young

A song that reflects my feeling about Danny is "Forever Young," written by Bob Dylan and performed by various artists over the years. Its lyrics are full of blessings, as Danny's life was. Danny wrote that "We are all so young, if not in body at least at heart." Danny's friend Sam Julian added art to the words that follow these:

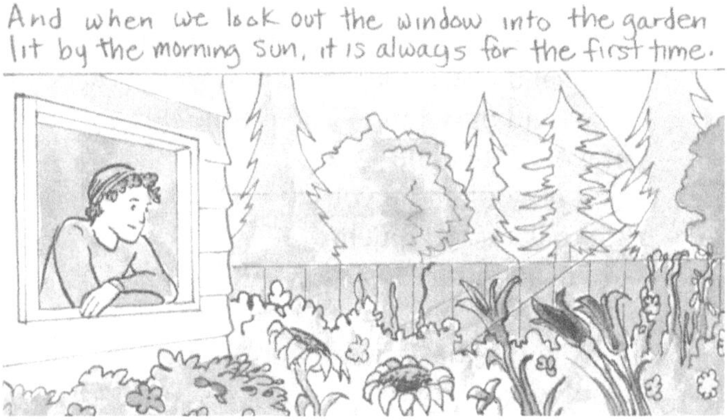

The Irish singer /songwriter Phil Coulter's inspiring verse places "forever young" in this story's context:

> You have nothing to fear from death,
> For only in death will you be forever young.
> Once again you will be with your loved ones
> And together your will dance and sing.
> Together you will dance and sing.
> Together you will dance and sing.

32
The Tenth Year Remembrance

While Danny died on October 31, 2007, the best day to have a tenth year remembrance of his life was a few days before on Saturday, October 28, 2017. We had a wonderful event with lots of family, friends, music, pictures, tributes, and shared memories that blended into a wonderful celebration of Danny's love, life, and light.

The gathering took place at ARTS, A Reason to Survive, mentioned before ,a non-profit located in National City, just south of San Diego, California.

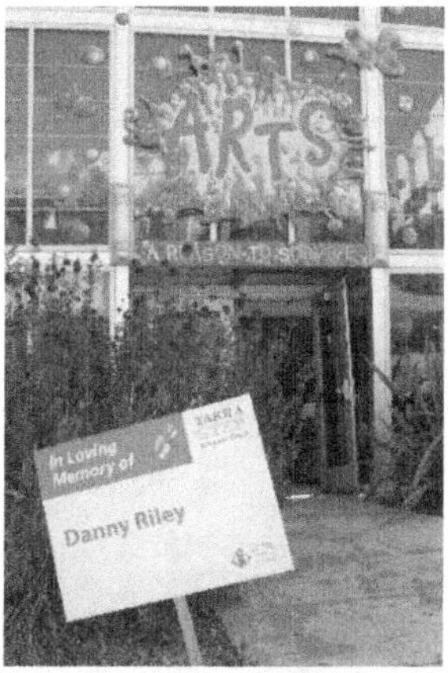

We took over all the rooms, especially the main hall and transformed it into a lively mix of musical presentations, one of which was a filmed-interpretative dance to Danny's song "Mountain's Edge," readings, shared memories, and touching moments, culminating with a video of Danny practicing his favorite song: Leonard Cohen's "Hallelujah."

The lobby were lined with photo boards of Danny and the large room off the main entrance had exhibits related to Danny's life and the ways he has been remembered over the last ten years for people to view, as they listened to a wonderful pianist.

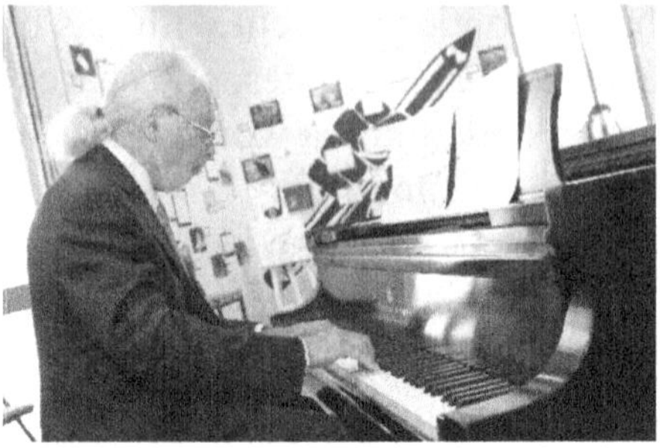

Danny's guitar which Jack Johnson had a display at all of his concerts on the 2008 tour.

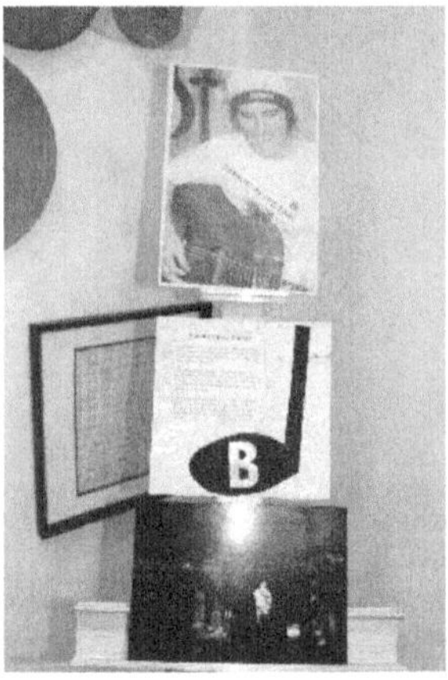

However, it was in the big hall where the main activities of the day took place. Good food, lavations, and a joyful spirit combined to make a memorable day. One performer after another took the stage to share a song, a memory or a special sentiment for or about Danny.

Jacob Tell, Danny's cousin. Alicia set the tone by saying over the last The emcees were Alicia Riley, Danny's sister, and ten years we have all changed but the memories of Danny's laughter, love of music, a good story and the closeness of family and friends were still strong, evidenced by so many present and actively sharing in the celebration.

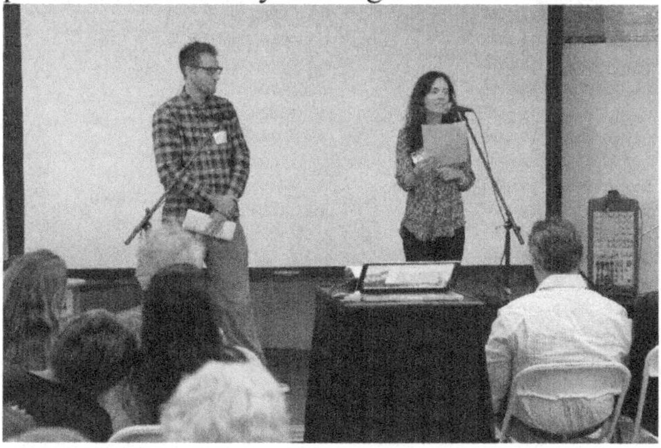

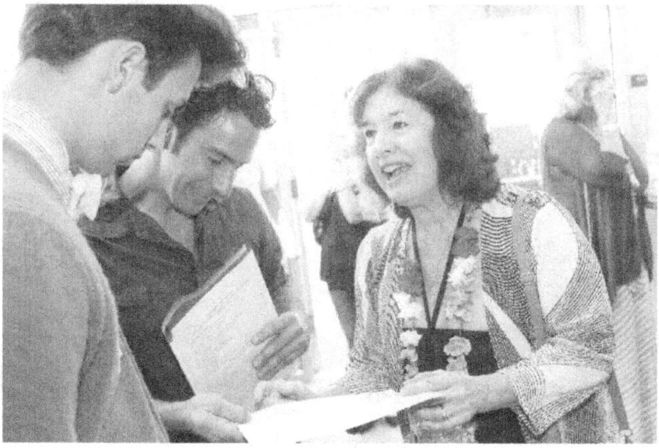

Maggi chatting with Matt and his son Ben

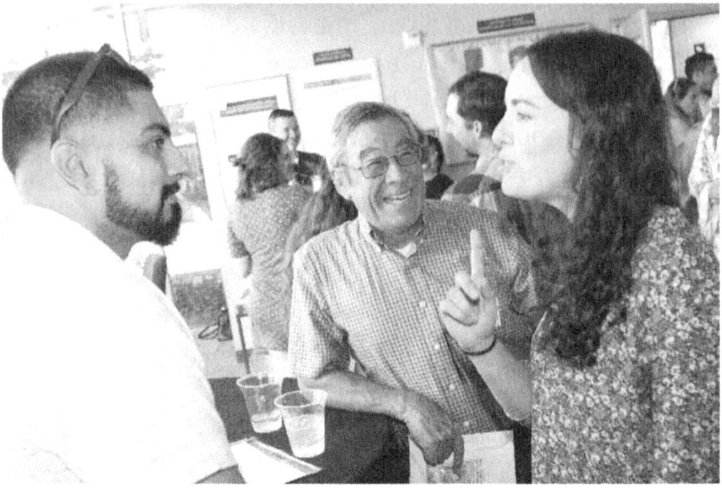

Alicia chatting with a former teammate and a soccer coach of Danny.

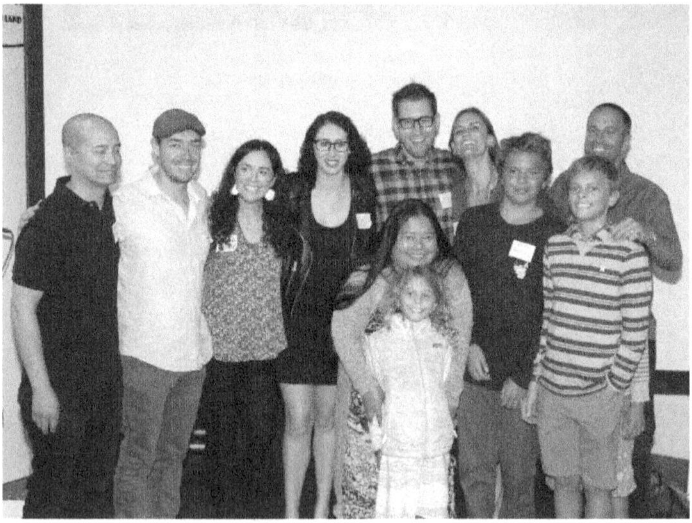

Danny's cousins on the Baker-side

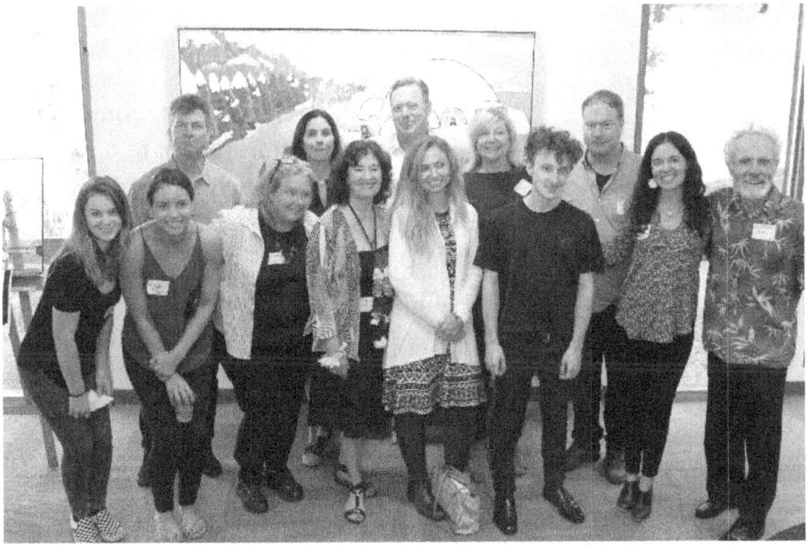

Members of the Riley clan

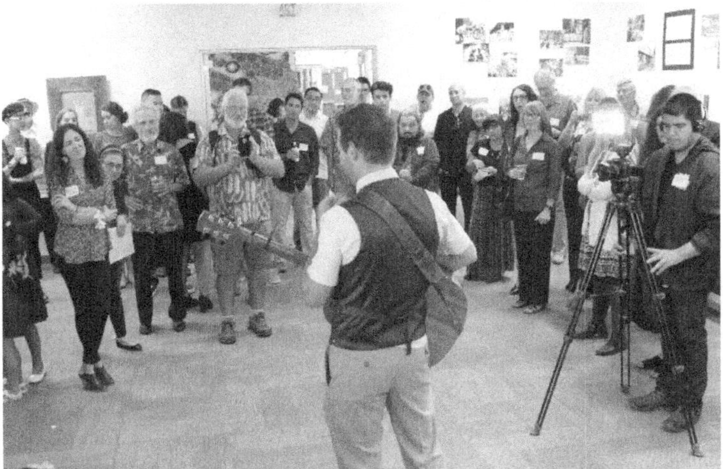

Singer/songwriter and good friend Michael Tiernan

Postscript

As I wrote in the "Build Up," I hoped this would be a good story, one that would bring readers to appreciate the stories that the joys and sorrows their lives inspire. While the words and pictures are about Danny Riley, most of the pieces that make up the mosaic can be found in any family who has faced challenges and felt the support of family, friends, and others who share their journey.

Danny loved a good story or joke. The picture below of Danny with his cousins Sheila and Rowan, listening to one of my stories, was taken in late August 2007 after his third brain surgery.

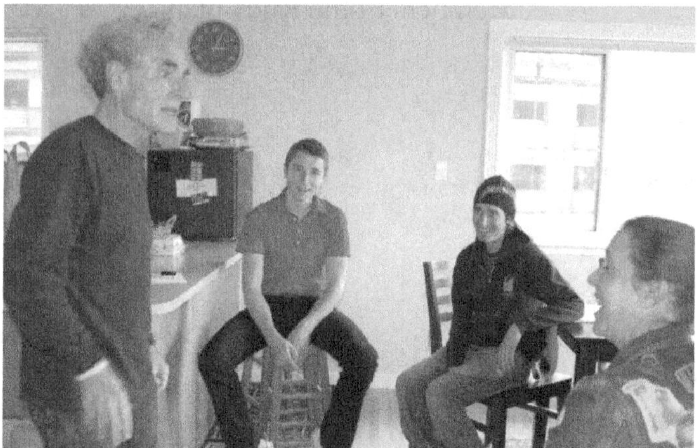

If a picture is worth a thousand words then this one shouts out that the smiles of life can brighten the hardest times. Even the toughest challenges can spark good stories, ones that enrich our lives and deepen our appreciation of the gifts we share on life's journey.

Danny wrote many songs and even described what a "good song" should contain:

> a good song captures something real. it can be anything. any emotion. any moment. any image. just as long as its real. or not. but that its honest. and tangible. thats what music is. the expression of things in a form we can understand on a different level.

I have a sense Danny would think this is a "good story" because it about something real, emotional, and honest: his journey with brain cancer, filled with music, family, friends, courage, pain, and hope.

And if my parting has left a void,
Then fill it with remember joy:
Friendship shared, a laugh, a kiss…
Ah yes, these things I, too, shall miss.
My life's been full, I've savored much:
Good times, good friends, a loved-one's touch.
Perhaps my time seemed all too brief—
Don't shorten yours with undue grief.
Be not burdened with the tears of sorrow,
Enjoy the sunshine of the morrow.

Remembered Joy-An Irish Poem

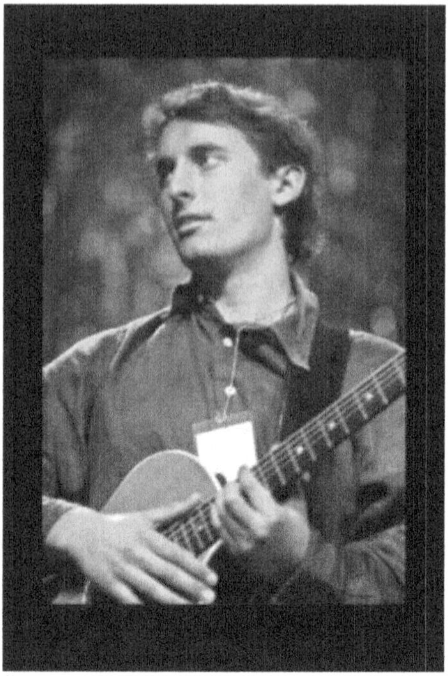

"oh but you havent shut me up yet!
ive got a new life
ive left all the strife
tucked in beneath ragged sheets,
sleeping on weathered pillows.
for those forgotten dreams
there is a fresh new window,
to gaze through
on rainy days,
and lonely days.
this is the beauty.
this is the new life."

-Danny Riley

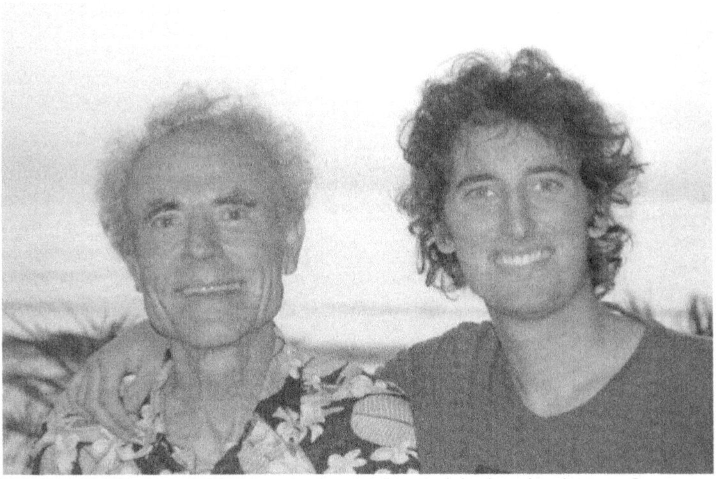

Frank and Danny Riley in August 2007 with the horizon of the Pacific Ocean in the background. Two months later, Danny crossed his final horizon leaving his light to color life like a beautiful sunset.

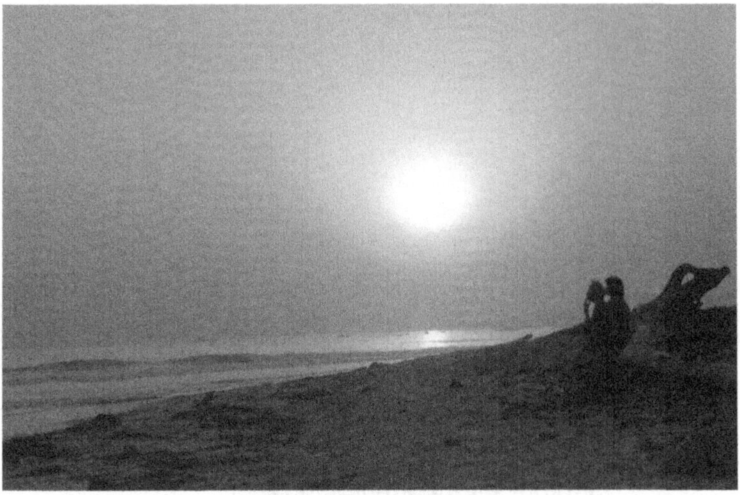

Made in the USA
Monee, IL
04 November 2026

67379627R00105